Additional Ac  ;

"Dr. Cozolino has set the groundwork for what will become the new standard of treatment in psychology and in functional neurologic conditions. In this book, he takes his foundational work to the next level; he not only defines in neurological terms what is happening in the brain of those who seek therapy, but he now also explains how therapy actually affects the brain and the nervous system—and therefore how it actually works. This is a must read for every clinician."

—Dr. Robert Melillo,
author of *Neurobehavioral Disorders of Childhood: An Evolutionary Perspective* and *Disconnected Kids*, President Emeritus of the International Association of Functional Neurology and Rehabilitation

"In *Why Therapy Works*, Louis Cozolino leads us through his personal journey to answer the question of what principles underlie successful psychotherapy. This readable and accessible book insightfully explains that therapies work as the therapist moves the client between feelings and thoughts, between implicit memories and explicit expressions, until the client diffuses the power of the implicit feelings. This dynamic process puts meaning and words to the often unbounded feelings that promote states of helplessness, frustration, anxiety, and despair."

—Stephen Porges,
PhD, author of *The Polyvagal Theory*, Distinguished University Research Scientist at Indiana University

About The Author

Lou Cozolino, PhD, is a writer, professor, and practicing psychologist in Los Angeles, California. In addition to holding degrees in philosophy, theology, and clinical psychology from Harvard and UCLA, he has worked and written in the areas of neuroscience, neuropsychiatry, and education. His clinical interests focus on the recovery from dysfunctional families, childhood trauma, and head injuries, using a combination of psychodynamic and systems approach informed by neurobiology.

Lou lectures around the world on attachment, brain development, evolution, and the synthesis of neuroscience and psychotherapy. In addition to *Why Therapy Works*, he is the author of *The Neuroscience of Psychotherapy 2e*, *The Making of a Therapist*, *The Neuroscience of Human Relationships 2e*, *The Healthy Aging Brain*, *The Social Neuroscience of Education*, and *Attachment-Based Teaching*. He has also written shorter pieces on child abuse, schizophrenia, language, and cognition. His current interests are in the area of the application of neuroscience and evolution to education and leadership. He is series editor for the Norton Series on Interpersonal Neurobiology and the Norton Series on the Social Neuroscience of Education.

Why Therapy Works

USING OUR MINDS TO CHANGE OUR BRAINS

Louis Cozolino

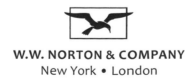

W.W. NORTON & COMPANY
New York • London

For information abut permission to reproduce selections from this
book, write to Permissions, W. W. Norton & Company, Inc.,
500 Fifth Avenue, New York, NY 10110

For information about special discounts for bulk purchases,
please contact W. W. Norton Special Sales at
specialsales@wwnorton.com or 800-233-4830

Manufacturing by Maple Press
Production manager: Christine Critelli

Library of Congress Cataloging-in-Publication Data

Cozolino, Louis J.
Why therapy works : using our minds to change our brains /
Louis Cozolino. — First edition.
pages cm
Includes bibliographical references and index.
ISBN 978-0-393-70905-6 (hardcover)
1. Psychotherapy. 2. Evidence-based medicine. I. Title.
RC480.5.C647 2016
616.89—dc23
2015024262

W. W. Norton & Company, Inc.
500 Fifth Avenue, New York, N.Y. 10110
www.wwnorton.com

W. W. Norton & Company Ltd.
Castle House, 75/76 Wells Street, London W1T 3QT

1 2 3 4 5 6 7 8 9 0

*This book is dedicated to Lennart Heimer,
a great man and a wonderful teacher.*

Contents

Part Three
DISSOCIATION AND INTEGRATION: APPLICATIONS TO PSYCHOTHERAPY

Acknowledgments

I WOULD LIKE to thank Deborah Malmud and the folks of W. W. Norton for their guidance, support, and hard work in the creation of this book. Thanks also to my colleagues at Pepperdine University, especially Vanessa Davis for her enthusiastic contribution to this effort. I would like to express my gratitude to my Interpersonal Neurobiology family for their kindness, commitment to healing others, and their support for one another, including Bonnie Badenoch, Bonnie Goldstein, Kyra Haglund, Richard Hill, Pat Ogden, Jaak Panksepp, Debra Pearce-McCall, Allan Schore, Dan Siegel, Marion Solomon, Stan Tatkin, and Bessel van der Kolk. A very special thanks goes to Erin Santos who, with great patience and attention to detail, oversaw all aspects of this book, contributed many valuable ideas, and smiled all the way. And finally, thanks to Susan and Sam for warming my heart at the start of each day.

Preface

AFTER A DOZEN years in school, thousands of hours of supervision, and a mountain of reading, I finally began a psychotherapy practice. Although still woefully unprepared, I tried to act like I knew what I was doing. Of course, it wasn't long before a new client, a no-nonsense businessman, asked this simple, straightforward question: "How does this psychotherapy business work?"

So I began to tell him about the scheduling, fees, cancellation policy, and so on. "No," he interrupted, "not those things. How does psychotherapy actually make you better?"

I apologized for misunderstanding his question and told him that we would first build our relationship, that he would be as open and honest as he could, and that we would work together to uncover unconscious issues. After that we would create experiments in the world to expand his emotional and behavioral repertoires. As I was speaking, I could see that he was getting frustrated, but he decided to try one more time. "No. I know all about the how-to's of therapy." He searched his brain for a different set of words and finally asked a question that has been on my mind ever since.

"What are the mechanisms of action? How will doing these things lead to the changes I need to make?"

I replied, "Great question!" as I searched my mind for an answer, assuming I had one somewhere. What I had were explanations from a dozen different therapeutic modalities I had been trained in. I thought of explaining why therapy worked in the language of systems theory, object relations, and Cognitive-Behavioral Therapy—then stopped myself. I remembered that I had never been completely satisfied with any of these explanations, and somewhere along the way I had given up looking for one. My stumbling answer undermined his confidence in me and my confidence in myself. In that moment, I realized that I needed to find a rational explanation, a mechanism of action beyond the usual therapeutic philosophies and metaphors.

That psychotherapy works was a basic assumption of my training, and all of my training was focused on how to practice. Like monks and soldiers, therapists of all denominations assume that god is on their side. The various forms of psychotherapy were built on experience—what works and what doesn't work. And while I learned how to administer treatments, I had never found a satisfactory explanation for why they worked. A lot of it seemed to rest on faith.

I was confident that each form of psychotherapy I had studied had the potential to help a group of clients to overcome their symptoms and achieve higher levels of functioning, happiness, and insight. I also saw that the sectarianism of the therapeutic schools limited our understanding of the underlying curative elements of psychotherapy.

I came to believe that in order to understand how psychotherapy works, we have to start from the bottom up, beginning with the brain, how it evolved, and especially how it evolved to learn, unlearn, and relearn. We need to understand how the brain responds to stress and how that response can result in symptoms and suffering. We also have to recognize that the brain is a social organ and that we can leverage the power of human relationships to regulate anxiety and stimulate learning.

If the same client came to me today and asked why therapy works, I still wouldn't have a perfect answer. I would, however, be able to construct an explanation with a scientific foundation that cuts across the countless types of treatment. And while science is, in many ways, just another metaphor, it provides a nonshaming explanation for human struggles and the mechanisms of action of the therapeutic process. Some of these ideas may even help us expand our case conceptualizations to include brain functioning and to more deeply appreciate the value of multidisciplinary collaborations.

This book is divided into three sections. The first, *The Thinking Brain: Consciousness and Self-Awareness*, lays a broad scientific framework for how evolution sets us up for mental distress while also providing us with the tools to heal each other. I describe why we have to look beyond words, diagnoses, and presenting problems to the deep history of our species and the inner histories of each of our clients to discover the paths to positive change.

The second section, *The Social Brain: Embodied and Embedded*, focuses on how our brains evolved into social organs and how our interpersonal lives are a source of both pain and power. I explore how our brains are programmed to connect in intimate relationships through the study of attachment schema and programmed to behave in groups via social status schema. I do my best to make the case for the centrality of attachment and social status for both health and illness. The text also explores core shame, an outgrowth of primitive instincts that enforce group cooperation, coordination, and control. Then I attempt to demonstrate the significance of shame management for healthy function and to fulfill the goals of therapy that help us be better able to love and work.

In the third and final section, *Dissociation and Integration: Applications to Psychotherapy*, I focus on the mechanisms and effects of anxiety, stress, and trauma. A central theme of the work we do is healing the impact of negative experiences on the brain, mind, and relationships. An important distinction is drawn between brief stressors and the early chronic stress often experienced by our most challenging clients. I then focus on the importance of narratives to self-regulation, neural integration, and positive change. I conclude by touching on some basic philosophical ideas from Buddhism that have helped me incorporate diverse perspectives from multiple fields, including the sciences and humanities.

In order to discover the processes underlying therapeutic change, we have to look beyond and below the particulars of specific forms of therapy to the commonalities of human evolution, biology, and experience. The answers to the question of why therapy works are embedded in the underlying mechanisms of adaptation and change within our brains, minds, and relationships.

WHY THERAPY WORKS

PART ONE

The Thinking Brain

Consciousness and Self-Awareness

CHAPTER 1

Why Humans Need Therapy

Evolution is a problem-creating as well as a problem-solving process.
Jonas Salk

IF NECESSITY IS the mother of invention, then what necessities gave rise to the invention of psychotherapy? The answer to this question lies in our evolutionary history and how it is expressed in our biology, relationships, and day-to-day experiences. While evolution is a process of adaptation, each adaptation leads to new challenges for which new adaptations need to arise. As most of us have experienced, things that seemed like a good idea initially can have unforeseen consequences and prove to be problematic down the road.

The human mind is made up of a tapestry of genetics, biology, and relationships that allow us to be interwoven into the superorganisms we call families, tribes, and cultures. Our deep evolutionary history accounts for the profound connections among our bodies, minds, and the nature and quality of our relationships. It has also provided us with the ability to heal others in psychotherapy.

Anatomically, modern humans evolved from our primate ancestors around 100,000 years ago. It seems to have taken another 50,000 years for our brains and cultures to evolve sufficient complexity to make us capable of language, planning, and creativity. But alas, this very complexity led to new challenges. The more recently emergent powers of logic, imagination, and empathy are built upon primitive mammalian and reptilian networks that drive our fears, superstitions, and prejudices. Coordinating scores of neural systems from different stages of evolution creates such a high level of complexity that our brains are extremely vulnerable to dysregulation, dissociation, and errors in thinking and judgment.

The artifacts of human prehistory displayed in museums, such as skulls, jewelry, and stone tools, pale in comparison to those inside our heads. Through a million years of conservation, innovation, and mutation, our brains have become a patchwork of old and new systems, many with different languages, operating systems, and processing speeds. At each point in our evolution, survival-based selections were made, allowing our species to adapt to new challenges. These adaptations also set the stage for new problems to arise in the future. Alas, evolution is not a strategic plan for the future but an adaptation to present conditions.

Here are several evolutionary artifacts that account for much of the psychological distress that brings us and our clients to psychotherapy. Although they are divided here for the purposes of definition, you will soon realize that these aspects of brain functioning are interdependent and mutually reinforcing. These core principles serve as the conceptual foundation for the chapters ahead.

Evolutionary Strategies That Result in Psychological Stress

#1 *The Vital Half Second*

> *Man is an over-complicated organism who may die out for want of simplicity.*
>
> Ezra Pound

As Freud, Charcot, and many before them recognized, our brains have multiple parallel tracks for processing conscious and unconscious information. The first is a set of early evolving, fast systems for our senses, motor movements, and bodily processes that we share with other animals. These primitive systems, which are nonverbal and inaccessible to conscious reflection, are referred to as implicit memory, the unconscious, or somatic memory. These are the memories that we do not consciously remember, but never forget. These fast systems are likely all that our ancestors had until the recent emergence of conscious awareness.

The later-evolving systems involved in conscious awareness, also called the slow systems, eventually gave rise to narratives, imagination, and abstract thought. This slow system, which developed as a result of complex social interactions and the larger brains they require, gave rise to self-awareness and self-reflection. The difference in processing speed between the fast and slow systems is approximately one half second. This vital half second is one of the primary reasons that we need psychotherapy. Let me explain.

A half second may not seem like much, but it is a long time for the brain. While it takes 500–600 milliseconds (half a second) for brain activity to register in conscious awareness, our brains process sensory, motor, and emotional information in 10–50 milliseconds. This is because conscious processing requires the participation of so many more neurons and neural systems. Evidence of the activity of the fast system is with us every day. If we touch a hot stove or are cut off while driving, our bodies react faster than conscious awareness. This is difficult to comprehend because our minds also construct the illusion that we are in conscious control of these reflexes.

Although a half second is a long time in terms of neural communication, it is barely perceptible to conscious awareness. During this vital half second, our brains work like search engines, unconsciously scanning our memories, bodies, and emotions for relevant information. In fact, 90% of the input to the cortex comes from internal neural processing, not the outside world. This half second gives our brains the opportunity to construct our present experience based on a template from the past that our minds view as objective reality. The result is that we feel like we are living in the present moment when, in reality, we live half a second behind. The processing gap between the two systems also helps us to understand why so many of us continue in old, ineffective patterns of behavior despite repeated failures.

By the time we become consciously aware of an experience, it has already been processed many times, activated memories, and initiated complex patterns of behavior. Examples of this process are attachment schema and transference, where the brain uses past relationships to shape our perceptions of the thoughts, feelings, and intentions of others. Distortions embedded within this projective process can damage a lifetime of relationships without us ever being aware that it is taking place. The fact that so much of our conscious experience is based on unconscious brain processing makes us extremely vulnerable to misperceptions and misinformation that our minds assume to be true. The greater the distortions, the more difficult it is to successfully love and work. Making the unconscious conscious was Freud's primary goal, while correcting biases in implicit processing is at the heart of Cognitive-Behavioral Therapy. All therapies attempt to address the processing biases created by the vital half second in their own way.

#2 The Primacy of Early Learning

> *There is no present or future, only the past happening*
> *over and over again, now.*
> Eugene O'Neill

Not only did the fast systems evolve first, but they also develop first during childhood. These fast systems learn, remember, and influence how our brains and minds construct conscious experience for the rest of our lives. Because remembering what we learn is a function of the later-developing slow systems, we don't consciously remember what we learned as infants and young children. This is one of the reasons why early learning has such a powerful influence on us throughout our lives. Psychotherapy is an opportunity to do some mental time travel to find out what we learned as young children and to learn the enduring effects that these lessons have had on us.

Even before birth, primitive regions of our brains are deeply affected by our biological, social, and emotional experiences. In fact, much of our most important learning occurs during our first few years of life when our primitive brains are in control. For example, the amygdala (our executive center for fear processing) is fully mature by eight months of gestation. The amygdala also happens to be a central component in the development of our attachment and social status schema, our ability to regulate our emotions, and our sense of self-worth. On the other hand, the cortical networks that will come to regulate and inhibit the amygdala will take two decades or more to mature.

The fact that so much learning occurs at the beginning of life is one of nature's standard operating procedures. In the womb, the child's biology is shaped by the mother's day-to-day experiences. After birth, the brain is shaped by the baby's interactions with the mother, other caretakers, and the physical environment. This strategy allows each human brain to adapt to a very specific environment. Culture, language, climate, nutrition, and parents, factors that may differ radically from culture to culture, generation to generation, and even day to day, shape each of our brains in unique ways. This is highly adaptive because, unlike most animals, every human baby can learn to fit in to whatever physical and social environment he or she is born into.

Because the first few years of life are a period of exuberant brain development, early experience has a disproportionate impact on the development of the brain's information super-highways. Parents' nonverbal communications and patterns of responding to the infant's basic needs shape the baby's brain and how the baby perceives the world. In good times and with good enough parents, this early brain building will serve the child well throughout life. The bad news comes when factors are not so favorable, such as in the case of parental psychopathology, where the brain may be sculpted in ways that later become maladaptive.

Misattuned parents, brutal social systems, war, and prejudice can have a tremendous impact on early brain development. For most of us, these memories remain forever inaccessible to conscious consideration or modification. We mature into self-awareness years later, having been programmed by early experiences with feelings, perceptions, and beliefs that we automatically assume to be true. In the absence of an ability to consciously connect our feelings and thoughts to past experiences, our negative feelings and behaviors seem to arise without cause from within. We are left to make sense of our confusion, fear, and pain with negative attributions about ourselves and the world based on biased and inadequate information.

As adolescents and adults, we seek therapy because we find ourselves unable to form meaningful relationships, manage our emotions, or feel worthy of love. The reasons for our struggles often remain buried in networks of implicit memory, inaccessible to conscious reflection. Psychotherapy guides us in a safe exploration of our early experiences and helps us create a narrative that associates these early experiences with the ways in which our brains and minds distort our current lives. In the process, our symptoms come to be understood as forms of implicit memory instead of insanity, character pathology, or plain stupidity. This process can open the door to greater compassion for oneself, openness to others, and the possibility for healing.

#3 Core Shame

> *Nothing you have done is wrong, and nothing you can do can*
> *make up for it.*
> Gershen Kaufman

The experience of shame is a central aspect of early social and emotional learning. Core shame needs to be differentiated from appropriate shame and guilt that emerge later in child-hood. Appropriate shame is an adaption to social behavior required by the group. Core shame, on the other hand, is an instinctual judgment about the self, and it results in a sense of worthlessness, a fear of being found out, and a desperate striv-ing for perfection. In essence, core shame is tied to our primi-tive instinct to be a worthy part of the tribe; it is a failure to internalize a deep sense of bonded belonging. As a result, peo-ple with core shame feel damaged, unlovable, and abandoned. Thus, core shame becomes a central factor in the perpetuation of insecure attachment and social status schema.

During the first year of life, parent-child interactions are mainly positive, affectionate, and playful. As infants grow into toddlers, their increasing motor abilities, impulsivity, and exploratory urges lead them to plunge headfirst into danger. The unconditional affection of the first year gives way to loud exclamations of "No," "Don't," "Stop" and a shift in the use of the child's name from a term of affection to a command or warning. This parent-to-child warning mechanism, seen in many animals, is designed to make children freeze in their tracks in order to protect them from predators and other dan-gers. This freeze response is reflected within the autonomic nervous system by a rapid transition from sympathetic curiosity to parasympathetic inhibition. Experientially, children are snapped from a mode of exploration to a startled freeze. As a result, the child stops, looks downward, hangs his head, and rounds his shoulders.

This state of submissive inhibition is the same as when a dog hunches over, pulls his tail between his legs, and slinks away after being scolded. Similar postures occur in reaction to social exclusion, helplessness, and submission in virtually all social animals. It is nature's way of expressing what an adult might articulate by saying, "Please don't hurt me" or "Okay, you're the boss." But for many children, this rapid shift from sympathetic exploration to parasympathetic withdrawal is internalized as "I'm not lovable," and "my membership in the family is in question," both of which are life threatening to a child, whose survival depends upon unconditional acceptance.

A parallel to these experiences may occur in early attachment relationships when a child's excited expectation of connection is met with indifference, disapproval, or anger from a parent or caretaker. This misattunement in the attachment relationship likely triggers the same rapid shift from sympathetic to parasympathetic dominance, and it is translated by the developing psyche as shame, rejection, and abandonment.

Differences in temperament or personality between parent and child and the resulting misattunement can contribute to the development of core shame. In other families, parents who were abandoned, neglected, or abused as children may use shaming, criticism, and sarcasm as a predominant parenting style with their own children. This is quite common among rigid and authoritarian parents, religious cults, military families, or when there is mental illness or unresolved trauma in one or both parents.

What began as a survival strategy to protect our young has become part of the biological infrastructure of later-evolving psychological processes related to attachment, safety, and self-worth. This is why the fundamental question "Am I safe?" has become interwoven with the question "Am I lovable?" With core shame, the answer is a painful "No!" As a result, people with core shame often have difficulty taking risks, choose abusive or nonsupportive partners, and cannot tolerate being alone. Although core shame may not be cured, therapy gives clients the skills to reality test their maladaptive beliefs, behaviors, and emotions.

#4 The Anxiety Bias and the Suppression of Language Under Stress

> *Evolution favors an anxious gene.*
> Aaron Beck

The prime directive of survival for every living thing, from single-cell organisms to human beings, is to approach what sustains life while avoiding what puts us at risk. The better and faster a species is at discerning between the two, the more likely it is to survive. Reptiles evolved a structure called the amygdala that has been conserved in later-evolving mammals, primates, and humans. The primary job of the amygdala is to appraise the desirability or danger of things in our world and to motivate us to move toward or away depending on its decision.

When the amygdala becomes aware of danger, it sends sig- ls to the autonomic nervous system to prepare to fight or ee. Half a second later, we consciously experience anything om anxiety to panic. Some things that trigger fear signals in the amygdala, such as snakes and heights, appear to be hardwired, genetic memories that harken back to our tree-dwelling ancestors. Others are learned associations based on experience that are activated during the vital half second that can make us avoid dogs, public speaking, or intimacy.

It appears that evolution has shaped our brains to err on the side of caution whenever it might be remotely useful. Not such a bad idea for prey animals in the wild, but a really bad idea for humans. We have really big brains that create large societies filled with complexity and stress. The amygdala reacts to traffic jams, the thought of asteroids hitting the earth, or getting a B on an exam as threats to life and limb, a design flaw that provides psychotherapists with an abundance of job security.

Fear inhibits executive functioning, problem-solving abilities, and emotional regulation. In other words, fear makes us rigid, inflexible, and dumb. We become afraid of taking risks and learning new things, leading us to remain in dysfunctional patterns of behavior, to hold onto failed strategies, and to remain in destructive relationships. The amygdala seems to use survival as vindication of its strategy, leading the agoraphobic to assume, "I haven't set foot outside my house in 10 years, and I'm still alive, which *must* be because I haven't set foot outside my house in 10 years." The amygdala's job is to keep us alive, and it has the neural authority to veto happiness and well-being for the sake of survival. Psychotherapy has to break into this closed logical loop by interrupting the cycle of dysfunctional thinking and reinforcement.

When animals hear a loud or threatening sound, they startle, freeze in their tracks, scan the environment for danger, and become silent. The logic is quite clear—avoid detection, locate the source of danger, and respond. These ancient responses, along with the structures that support them, have been conserved in humans. During high states of arousal, the brain area responsible for expressive speech (Broca's area) becomes inhibited. This may explain a variety of human phenomena, from becoming tongue-tied when talking to the boss to the speechless terror associated with trauma.

While the momentary inhibition of sound production may have no negative consequences for other animals, it can be disastrous for humans. For us, shutting down sound means losing the language we need in order to connect with others and to organize our conscious experiences. Language serves the integration of neural networks of emotion and cognition that supports emotional regulation and attachment. Putting feelings into words and constructing narratives of our experiences make an invaluable contribution to a coherent sense of self.

Central tenets of psychotherapy include expressing the unexpressed, making the unconscious conscious, and integrating thoughts and feelings. Experiences that occur before we develop speech or in the context of trauma remain unintegrated and isolated in dissociated neural networks. By stimulating Broca's area, connecting words with feelings, and helping clients to construct a coherent narrative of their experiences, we help restore a sense of perspective and agency and an ability to edit dysfunctional life stories. Language has evolved to connect us to each other and to ourselves, a primary reason for the success of the talking cure.

#5 *Illusion*

> *We do not live to think. . . . We think in order that we*
> *may succeed in surviving.*
>
> José Ortega y Gasset

Our minds are masters of illusion. Highly dedicated psycho-analysts, neuroscientists, and Zen Buddhists have spent their lives trying to penetrate these illusions in order to discern the nature of reality. However, using an illusion generator to see beyond illusions has its limitations. While much still remains a mystery, one thing is clear—conscious experience is full of distortions. While many of these distortions are designed to enhance survival, they also make us vulnerable to many forms of suffering that bring people to psychotherapy.

Defense mechanisms and all of the attribution biases discovered by social psychology provide ample proof that our thinking is biased in self-favorable and anxiety-reducing ways. In fact, it has often been suggested that depression results from perceiving reality too accurately—a sort of denial deficit disorder. Groupthink, halo effects, and humor also grease the social wheels, allowing us to put a positive spin on the behavior of our family and friends.

While self-deception decreases anxiety, it also increases the likelihood that we will successfully deceive others. If we believe our self-deceptions, we are less likely to give away our real thoughts and intentions via nonverbal signs and behaviors. Reaction formation, or behaviors and feelings that are opposite to our true desires, are often quite effective in deceiving others. Thus, we are all naturally born con men, who first and foremost deceive ourselves.

In short, distortions of conscious awareness are not character flaws, but preprogrammed by-products of our evolutionary history based on their proven survival value. They help us to be strong, assertive, and confident in the face of threat. Our distortions allow us all to believe that we are above average and for two warring nations to both believe that god is on their side. The downside of these distortions comes when we have so much confidence in our point of view that we repeat the same dysfunctional behaviors in spite of all evidence to the contrary. The prevalence of illusions, distortions, and misperceptions is why reality testing is so important in almost all forms of therapy. The most naive observer, let alone a trained therapist, can see many things about us more clearly than we can see them ourselves. Questioning one's assumptions, internalizing interpretations, and learning about how the brain mismanages information are all potential roads to positive change.

As therapists, we attempt to provide our clients with alternative perspectives and new information in order to disrupt a closed and self-reinforcing logical system. And when therapy is at its most useful, clients are able to internalize perceptions and insights from others that improve their ability to test the reality of their experience beyond their habitual distortions. Psychotherapy provides us with an opportunity to make our unconscious conscious, creating a platform for the exploration of our maladaptive illusions.

CHAPTER 2

Why Therapy Works

The only person who is educated is the one who has learned how
to learn to change.
Carl Rogers

FORTUNATELY FOR US, the same evolutionary processes that gave rise to the sources of our emotional suffering also provided us with the tools to heal: our abilities to connect, attune, and empathize with others. Psychotherapy is not a modern intervention, but a relationship-based learning environment grounded in the history of our social brains. Thus, the roots of psychotherapy go back to mother-child bonding, attachment to family and friends, and the guidance of wise elders.

The potential success of therapy relies on three fundamental mechanisms of brain, mind, and relationships.

1. The brain is a social organ of adaptation, shaped by evolution to connect with and change through interactions with others. Psychotherapy leverages the ability of brains to attune and learn from one another in the service of adaptive change. This intimate interaction between human connection and learning has been forged over the eons in the crucible of social evolution.

2. Change depends upon the activation of neuroplastic processes. For any change to occur, our brains have to undergo structural changes that will be reflected in our thoughts, feelings, and behaviors. Thus, the success of psychotherapy depends upon the therapist's ability to stimulate neuroplasticity in the brains of clients—to make new connections, inhibit others, and link previously dissociated neural networks.

3. Together, we co-create narratives that support neural and psychic integration while creating a template to guide experience into the future. Through the co-construction of coherent self-stories, we are able to enhance our self-reflective capacity, creativity, and maturation. It is especially valuable in coming to understand our past, for the consolidation of identity, and to heal from trauma.

The Tools for Healing

#1 *The Social Brain*

> *Everything can be found in isolation except sanity.*
> Friedrich Nietzsche

An interesting thing happened during the evolution of our social brains. The primitive processes of neuroplasticity became interwoven with the more recently evolved aspects of sociality. In other words, the quality of attachment relationships has evolved to regulate neuroplasticity and learning. Secure attachment relationships support flexible, adaptive learning and higher-order executive functioning; insecure attachments support reactive behavior and rigid, trauma-based learning. This is why establishing a secure attachment within the therapeutic relationship serves as the matrix for positive change. So the essence of what we do as therapists is to connect with our clients in an exchange of emotions and information. Like neurons, we send and receive messages from one another across a synapse—the social synapse.

Definition: The Social Synapse

The social synapse is the space between us through which we communicate. The bandwidth of the social synapse includes both conscious and nonconscious modes of communication. On the surface we can point to gestures, words, and body language while unconscious forms of communication include pupil dilation, microfacial expressions, and odors.

To establish a bridge of attunement, we rely on many neural systems that receive and send social and emotional information. We use all of this information to create theories about what is on the minds of others. We establish internal representations of what is happening within them by simulating their internal states within us. We rely on attachment circuitry to establish bonds and to know how to apply the optimal balance of challenge and support to help our clients grow. We utilize all of the networks of our social brains in an attempt to articulate experiences that clients are presently unable to articulate themselves.

As discussed earlier, an important remnant of our evolutionary past, the amygdala, rests at the core of the brain. This ancient executive center has retained veto power over our modern cortical executive centers when it detects a threat. It is also like an elephant; it never forgets. The only chance we have at getting over a fear is to do what my grandfather suggested to me as a child: "Get back on the horse that threw you." This folk wisdom embodies the knowledge that fear becomes reinforced through avoidance and inhibited by confrontation. This is why a decrease in avoidance behavior is highly correlated with therapeutic success.

Approaching danger and surviving inhibits the amygdala's tendency to trigger the fight-flight response. Such situations can range from picking up a spider, to finishing the last class to get a degree, or going out on a first date. Risking new and seemingly dangerous experiments in the service of positive change requires a combination of courage, emotional support, and the ability to imagine success. Thus, successful therapists learn to be "amygdala whisperers" by leveraging the social brain in order to help clients face their fears in experiments that are developed collaboratively during sessions.

#2 Neuroplasticity

Plasticity . . . means the possession of a structure weak enough to yield to an influence, but strong enough not to yield all at once.
William James

Most generally, neuroplasticity refers to the birth, growth, development, and connectivity of neurons—the basic mechanisms of all learning. Existing neurons grow by connecting their projections (dendrites) during learning. Neurons interconnect to form neural networks, and neural networks, in turn, integrate with one another to perform increasingly complex tasks.

> ## Neuroscience Corner: Neuroplasticity
> Neuroplasticity is a general term that refers to any changes among, between, and within neurons as a result of learning or the natural processes of healthy development. It is the ability of the nervous system to change in response to experience and to encode that experience into its structure.

Because a brain is such a complicated government of systems, the possibilities of disconnections, misconnections, and failures of adaptation are almost endless. And because our brains depend so much on experience to help them develop properly, a lot can go wrong. When one or more neural networks necessary for optimal functioning remain undeveloped, unregulated, or unintegrated with others, we experience the complaints and symptoms for which we seek therapy.

We now assume that when psychotherapy results in symptom reduction or experiential change, the brain has, in some way, been altered: new connections have been made, dysfunctional systems altered or inhibited, or disconnected networks reintegrated. This suggests that all psychotherapists are neuroscientists who work to change the structure of the brain. Although the principles of plasticity have not been understood until recently, the practices and strategies of psychotherapy have been guided by their invisible hand since the beginning. Through trial and error, therapists have learned what works and what doesn't work, and we continue this work individually with our clients. What works is what optimizes plasticity and leads to positive change—we are all experimental neuroscientists.

Openness and trust are fragile creatures, even with the people we love most. The training of the therapist and the therapeutic context itself are designed to increase neuroplasticity in networks of the social brain to enhance support, trust, and availability. It turns out that a secure and positive therapeutic alliance generates a double neuroplastic punch. A positive emotional connection stimulates metabolic processes that activate plasticity while inhibiting stress.

Thus, safe and attuned connections create the possibility for both short-term and long-lasting modification of the brain. Through the security of a safe relationship, something new can be introduced into a previously closed and dysfunctional system. This is one of the ways in which relatives, friends, and tribe members enhance survival and lead to the emergence of culture. This is also why relationships are the most challenging aspect of life. Although there is endless debate about the relative merits of different forms of therapy, they all depend on the same underlying biopsychosocial-developmental mechanisms of change.

#3 Language, Storytelling, and Co-constructed Narratives

> *There is no greater agony than bearing an untold story inside you.*
> Maya Angelou

Human beings are natural storytellers, and the roots of the talking cure harken back to gatherings around ancient campfires. Through countless generations, we have shared stories of the hunt, the exploits of our ancestors, and morality tales of good and evil. The urge to tell stories and gossip is embedded in our psyches, wired into our brains, and woven into our DNA. This is why *People* magazine will always outsell *Scientific American*. For most of human history, oral communication and verbal memory were the repository of our collective knowledge. The drive of elders to repeatedly tell the same stories is matched only by the desire of young children to hear the same stories again and again. This lock-and-key information highway carries memories, ideas, and values across generations.

Stories also serve as powerful tools for neural network integration. The combination of a linear story line and visual imagery woven together with verbal and nonverbal expressions of emotion activates circuitry of both cerebral hemispheres, cortical and subcortical networks, the various regions of the frontal lobes, the hippocampus, and the amygdala. This integrative neural processing may also account, in part, for the positive correlations between coherent narratives and secure attachments. Further, shared stories contain images and ideas that stimulate imagination and link individuals to the group mind.

Narratives are also powerful because they allow us to have an objective distance on direct experience, creating the possibility of alternate viewpoints. Through stories, we can escape the emotions and influences of the moment and take time to reflect on our experience. We can also share versions of possible selves with others to receive input about our experiences and perspectives. Finally, we can experiment with new emotions, actions, and language as we edit the scripts of our lives.

Although it seems that children are little scientists discovering the world, we often miss that they are primarily engaged in discovering what the rest of us already know about them. As children we are told by others, and we gradually begin to tell others, who we are, what is important to us, and what we are capable of. This serves the continuity of culture from one generation to the next as parents reflexively strive to re-create themselves. This can be both good and bad depending on the parents and the goodness of fit with their children. Stories are powerful organizing forces that serve to perpetuate both healthy and unhealthy forms of self-identity. There is evidence that positive self-narratives aid in emotional security while minimizing the need for elaborate psychological defenses.

The role of language and narratives in neural integration, memory formation, and self-identity make them powerful tools in the creation and maintenance of the self. Putting feelings into words has long served a positive function for many individuals suffering from stress or trauma. Even writing about your experiences supports top-down modulation of emotion and bodily responses. In listening to our clients, we reflexively analyze their narratives for inaccurate, destructive, and missing elements. We then attempt to edit their narratives in a manner we feel would better support their adaptation and well-being.

#4 Self-Reflective Capacity

> The key to growth is the introduction of higher dimensions of consciousness into our awareness.
> Lao Tzu

Self-reflective capacity, the ability to think about our thoughts, feelings, and behaviors, has been found to correlate with both secure attachment and successful psychotherapy. This same ability has been called psychological mindedness by psychoanalysts and mindfulness in the self-help world. Self-awareness is derived from and reinforced by parents and therapists through the creation of narratives that include subjective states as objects of communication. We also come to learn that we are capable of evaluating old habits and attaining a more objective view of the expectations of others and the mandates of our childhoods. Therapy attempts to leverage this metacognitive vantage point to make new and more adaptive decisions.

The purpose of sharing our stories with others is to gain active participation in the co-construction of new narratives. Our own stories tend to become closed systems in need of new input. Therapists hope to teach their clients that not only can they edit their present story, but they can also be authors of new stories. With the aid of self-reflection, we help clients to become aware of narrative arcs of their life story and then help them understand that alternative story lines are possible. As the writing and editing processes proceed, new narrative arcs emerge along with the possibility of experimenting with more adaptive ways of thinking, feeling, and acting.

#5 Abstract Thought and Imagination

> *Imagination is more important than knowledge.*
> Albert Einstein

As the size of primate groups expanded, grooming, grunts, and hand gestures were gradually shaped into spoken language. Language made far more precise, complex, and subtle forms of communication possible. As social groups grew larger and language became more complex, more cortical space was required to process a greater amount of social information. This expanded topography was a contributing factor in the emergence of abstract thinking and imagination.

The human brain is characterized by the growth of an area called the inferior parietal cortex. This area, in collaboration with parts of the prefrontal cortex, appear to have allowed us to do three things that border on the miraculous. First, we are able to construct three-dimensional models of external objects in our imaginations. Second, we can manipulate and modify these models in our heads. Third, we can transform these objects of imagination into objects in the external world. We can apply our imagination, not only to external objects, but to ourselves.

Thus, humans are capable of imagining alternative selves, creating new narratives to become these selves, and then using narratives as blueprints for changing their lives. Countless blueprints are created and discarded during development as children and adolescents try on different identities. As we progress, we naturally outgrow old identities like a snake outgrows its skin. As we grow older, we often forget that we can change our stories, and we may become symptomatic when an old identity no longer fits who we've become.

Our imaginations allow us to escape the present moment, create alternative realities, and then begin our journey to find our new narratives. The hero's journey, found in the literature of every culture, is a reflection of an ancient drive to explore new worlds, which allowed early humans to survive and spread around the globe. As therapists, we can leverage this heroic instinct in the service of our clients to assist them in facing their fears and creating a new life story. This is the hero's journey of every culture—with shamans, medicine women, wise elders, and psychotherapists serving as guides.

Striving for Ignorance

Real knowledge is to know the extent of one's ignorance.
Confucius

We have yet to discover how the brain and mind construct consciousness. Our best guess is that conscious experience emerges through a convergence of sustained attention, working memory, learned behaviors, language, and culture. Because it's still a guess, all of us who work with or possess minds need to be humble about what we think we know. One thing that I am certain of is that I'm not certain of much, but I think I have some good working models.

As we saw earlier, conscious experience is constructed by the brain and mind in approximately half a second. Amazingly, this is enough time for the brain to use some portion of our 100 billion neurons and 100 trillion synaptic connections to construct a conscious perception. If 90% of brain activity is dedicated to internal processing, then only 10% is focused on figuring out what's going on in the external world. Natural selection has shaped conscious experience in the service of survival, so how we perceive things has been shaped to optimize our ability to live long enough to reproduce and protect our children. Remember—the way the brain and mind construct consciousness is dedicated to adaptation, not accuracy.

The brain is an organ of adaptation that predicts and controls outcomes in the service of survival. As such it has to learn from experience, organize automatic responses to all eventualities, and anticipate the future as fast as possible. This is why our perceptions are biased in the direction of making rapid decisions with minimal information. Whatever our decisions are, you may also notice that we tend to justify and rationalize our choices, even when we know they are wrong, to reduce ambiguity and uncertainty. The brain not only wants to make fast decisions, it wants us to act with certainty and congratulate ourselves, regardless of the outcome.

Using Our Minds to Change Our Brains

> *Shift happens.*
> Candace Perth

Why is it so hard for people to accept themselves? This is a complex question with a relatively simple answer. Our self-esteem, our ability to regulate our inner emotional world, and our comfort in relationships are all organized during the first year or two of life. During this time, there is a rapid down-loading of our mothers', fathers', and other caretakers' inner worlds into our implicit (unconscious) memory systems. Because we never remember learning any of these things, we come into self-consciousness later in life with most of our software already downloaded. Thus, we are full of emotions, reactions, and behaviors that we have to justify as we attempt to develop a coherent narrative about who we are as people.

We come to believe the narrative that we create, and we feel the need to be consistent with it even when it's a bad fit. If we have a narrative that doesn't fit us and we feel the instinctual need to adhere to it, we will inevitably become symptomatic. We seek therapy because of the symptoms (e.g., anxiety, depression, bad relationships), but we discover that the symptoms are the visible expressions of deeper issues. Our minds construct conscious experience based on three misperceptions: (1) we are experiencing the present moment; (2) we possess unlimited free will; and (3) we have access to accurate information about ourselves and the world. As you might imagine, the combination of these three illusions allows us to act with confidence and without hesitation. Let's examine these three beliefs.

Primates, including humans, possess brains with complex neural networks that become activated as we observe and interact with those around us. We have circuits that analyze the actions and gestures of others to develop a theory of mind—what others know, what their motivations may be, and what they might do next. This ability to intuit about what's on someone else's mind helps us predict their behavior—a capacity that supports group coordination and self-defense. We also have mirror neurons that link sensory, motor, and emotional brain networks to generate behaviors and feelings within us that mirror what is likely to be going on in those we are interacting with.

The existence of these mirror neurons and the theory of mind system reflects the fact that millions of years of evolution have been dedicated to refining systems for reading the emotions, thoughts, and intentions of others. We are quick to think we know others because these processes, and the attributions and emotions they trigger, are preconscious, automatic, and obligatory. All of this dedicated circuitry makes us very good at coming up with ideas about the motives and intentions of other people. It also allows us to learn through observation and practice new behaviors in our minds.

Neuroscience Corner: Mirror Neurons

Mirror neurons, located in the premotor regions of our frontal lobes, fire when we observe someone engaging in a specific behavior, such as saying a specific word or grasping an object. Some mirror neurons are so specific that they fire only when an object is grasped in a certain way by particular fingers. The same neurons also fire when we perform the action ourselves. Mirror neurons link observation and action, allowing us to (1) learn from others through observation; (2) anticipate and predict the actions of others, which supports group coordination and self-defense; and (3) activate emotional states supportive of emotional resonance and empathy.

Of course, there is an obvious downside to this ability as well—we are fairly prone to misreading ourselves. One reason is that while evolution has equipped us with awareness of others, it has not as yet seen fit to invest much in self-awareness and personal insight. This is probably why it is easy to see what is wrong with someone else, but difficult for us to see what is wrong with ourselves. In fact, the capacity to challenge our self-perceptions may have even been selected against during evolution because it can lead to self-doubt, hesitation, and demoralization. This may be why humans have unconscious mechanisms that distort reality in our favor.

In fact, we often project our own thoughts and feelings (which we may not recognize as our own) onto others and assume it is their truth, not our own. While Freud saw these projective processes as defensive, they may be a natural by-product of how our brains have evolved to process social information. Projection is automatic and lessens anxiety, while self-awareness can generate anxiety and requires sustained effort. Self-analysis is difficult because our inner logic is so interwoven with our natural reflex to avoid anxiety by blaming others.

The answer to the question of why therapy works can be addressed by asking another, more fundamental question: What do humans need? Beyond the basic survival needs of food and shelter, humans need to feel that they are accepted members of their groups. For a child, this is first the mother and later the father, siblings, and extended family. The need to be accepted gradually expands to include peers and romantic connections during adolescence and later to work, spouses, and children during adulthood. For social animals, connection is a fundamental drive, and our place within social groups is of central concern. Most people come to therapy because they don't feel accepted by others, and therefore, they don't accept themselves.

As Dr. Salk observed decades ago, evolution solves old problems and creates new ones. While a number of adaptative strategies created the need for psychotherapy, others have provided us with the tools to heal. The first is the power of secure relationships. The second is that we can leverage these relationships to stimulate neuroplasticity and brain growth. And the third is the ability of the body and the conscious mind to use self-awareness, stories, emotions, and bodily awareness to reshape neural circuitry in the service of improved adaptation. We are now capable of becoming aware of our misperceptions and working against our inherent biases to gain a clear perception of external reality. The good news is that our capacity to connect our minds with the minds of others allows us to counterbalance some of evolution's less than stellar decisions. The ability of brains and minds to attune and influence one another is at the heart of psychotherapy.

Neuroscience Corner: Genetics and Epigenetics

Our brains are built in the interface between experience and genetics, where nature and nurture become interwoven into a single process. Genes first serve as a template to organize the brain, activate relevant biological processes, and trigger sensitive periods of development. Genes then orchestrate the translation of experience into the structures of our brains through a process of transcription. Template genetics is the mechanism of action of the transmission of traits from one generation to the next. Transcription genetics is the translation of ongoing experience into the structure of the brain. Through transcription genetics, our experience becomes flesh, relationships shape the brain, and culture is passed across individuals and through time.

Since the discovery of the double helix in the 1950s, we have come to understand that the information that builds our brains and bodies is coded in four amino acid bases (adenine, thymine, guanine, and cytosine), which flow from DNA to messenger RNA to protein. Although this was a huge leap forward in our knowledge of the underlying processes of genetic transmission, it only accounts for about 2% of genetic expression. So what accounts for the other 98%?

This gets us back to the old nature-nurture debate: what do we inherit and what do we learn from experience? Our best guess is that almost everything involves an interaction between the two. While we inherit a template of genetic material (genotype), what gets expressed (phenotype) is guided by noncoded genetic information that is dependent on experience. Experience can include anything from toxic exposure to a good education; from high levels of sustained stress to a warm and loving environment; from feast to famine. An example of this process of particular relevance to emotional development and psychotherapy is the impact of early stress on the adult brain. Research with rats has demonstrated that early maternal deprivation downregulates the degree of neurogenesis and the response to stress during adulthood. Just as important for us, these processes are reversible later in life. As therapists, we attempt to reprogram these neural systems via a supportive relationship and the techniques we bring to bear during treatment. In other words, we are using epigenetics to change the brain in ways that enhance mental and physical well-being.

CHAPTER 3

The Nonpresenting Problem

Man is only fitfully committed to . . . thinking, seeing, learning,
knowing. Believing is what he is really proud of.
Martin Amis

IN CASE YOU haven't noticed, human thinking is deeply flawed. Not only that, but we are capable of holding onto our false beliefs for a lifetime in the face of considerable evidence to the contrary. Not only do people come to us for help, but they also put up a prolonged fight against accepting the assistance they pay us to provide. As a species, we humans can be dumb, stubborn, and proud—a costly combination.

While most therapists label a client's persistence in maintaining old behaviors, thoughts, and feelings as resistance, I believe that there is a better way to think about it. Our brains weave our experience of reality from millions of unconscious assumptions based on past learning. Interwoven with useful assumptions are those that can make our lives difficult or impossible. The problem is, our minds usually can't tell the difference.

Truth is, the brain doesn't care if our thinking makes sense; its main concern is to keep us alive. That's why it is willing to sacrifice evidence and logic for surviving another day. So what we usually call resistance may simply be primitive brain circuitry engaging in anxiety reduction by holding onto the beliefs that make us feel safe. As bad as your life may be, your amygdala pairs it with survival every moment you avoid death —change, even for the better, activates anxiety.

Although clients come to therapy for help, their primitive executive system—led by the amygdala—will go to great lengths to avoid change. Because the best defense is a good offense, clients will go so far as to try to convince us that they are fine and that we are the ones with the problem (this sometimes works because we really are the one with the problem). Because our brains are social organs and exert a strong influence over each other, clients sometimes convince us to see the world the way they do. This is not a sickness on their part or ours, just an aspect of having a social brain.

Hanging With the Primitive Brain

> *The greatest obstacle to discovery is not ignorance—*
> *it is the illusion of knowledge.*
> Daniel Boorstin

Therapists are like everyone else—we want to be powerful, successful, and influential, so it isn't always easy on us when a client's primitive brain outsmarts us and stalls treatment in a morass of confusing and contradictory beliefs. If you have been doing therapy for any amount of time, you have had this experience on a regular basis. This is what clients have to do on their way to healing; it is how the unconscious communicates. Despite this fact, it is quite common for therapists to feel discouraged, confused, and even angry with clients for making them feel frustrated and helpless. The risk is that some therapists abdicate responsibility for the treatment and spend the sessions daydreaming while clients fill the time with a litany of complaints, stories, or information. If this happens, your client's amygdala has won; you get paid, and the client stays safe and unchanged.

Clients come in with a complex web of beliefs, which you need to patiently explore and come to understand. The beliefs usually make complete sense to them and, like water to a fish, are often invisible. Because you swim in different waters, you will be able to see things that clients are blind to, but be careful what you reveal. We all need the water in our tanks to survive. The art of therapy includes the ability to gradually peel away layers of illusion in manageable portions. Fear is the enemy of psychological growth—the amygdala will see to that.

Should you find that you are bored while doing therapy, it is likely that you have been defeated by the client's need to avoid the problem. Think of your boredom as a signal that you have checked out and may be engaging in passive revenge for feeling incompetent. The only way out is to renew your therapeutic vows and go back into the fray. Look to the nonpresenting problem—what are they not saying? What feeling might the client be avoiding? What is behind all of the material being pushed forward? Look around the current issues to the deep history. Peer beyond thoughts and ideas to the core emotions such as fear, shame, and abandonment.

Diving Below the Surface

> *Data allow us to understand the past while a good theory*
> *helps us to predict the future.*
> Clayton Christensen

Presenting problems are clients' best guesses as to why they are sitting across from you. It is usually the event that has precipitated an emotional crisis, like the breakup of a relationship or the loss of a job. If clients have a little more insight, they may connect their current problem to life patterns they have come to recognize. As often as not, focusing on the presenting problem results in what has been described as a catastrophic comprehension of the psychic surface—catastrophic because the resources spent on therapy are wasted on issues that don't have the leverage to serve as mechanisms of change.

The primitive brain doesn't come into session and tell you what's wrong. First of all, the primitive brain is nonverbal, so it will communicate with you like an artist, through actions, emotions, and symbols. While your client might not be able to say that he has trouble expressing his hurt feelings to others, the primitive brain will create a sore throat or laryngitis. Your clients won't tell you that they resent that you have the power in the relationship, but they will tell you that your magazines are nerdy, that your furniture is out of style, or that your socks don't match (all of which have been said to me).

As new therapists, we are led astray early in training by being taught to focus on the presenting problem by answering questions such as, What brings the client to therapy? What does the client see as the problem? What will be the focus of our treatment? By what metric will we measure progress and treatment success?

There is a certain logic to this approach, especially when clients have an accurate idea of their problems. On the surface, we are providing a service; the client is the consumer, and his or her concerns should be the focus of our treatment. Clients are anxious about being in therapy, and inexperienced therapists are anxious because they don't have a clue what to do. Therefore, it is comforting for both parties to have a task that they can focus on. From the first minutes of therapy, both client and therapist are swept away in the busywork of filling out forms, checking off boxes, and coming to a rapid conclusion and solution.

Presenting problems almost always fall into three categories:

1. Symptoms: depression, anxiety, dissociation, etc.
2. Behaviors: self-harm, gambling, sarcasm, criticism, seduction, etc.
3. Relationships: conflicts, breakups, grief, loneliness, etc.

However, these presenting problems are most often the tip of the iceberg. Sometimes, symptoms are caused by underlying biochemical problems—like medication side effects or postpartum depression. But most often, a client's complaints point to the primary issues hidden below the surface. These are usually an array of genetic, historical, and experiential variables that bring clients to our office at a specific point in time. An eating disorder may reflect parental struggles for control, while depression could be the result of decades of chronic anxiety.

From its beginnings, psychotherapy has been all about looking beyond the information given. That is one of the things that separate therapists from friends, relatives, and other untrained people in our lives. A surgeon once told me that when he was asked to examine an X-ray and told to look at the left lung, he made it his lifelong practice to always look at the left lung last. He claimed that over the years he had discovered many other problems that he never would have seen if he only looked where he was told to look. Directions, he said, made him operate in a less intelligent manner—they actually directed his mind to miss things.

There is plenty of evidence that we miss significant things that are right in front of us if we are looking for something else. In an interesting study, researchers put a black-and-white drawing of a gorilla on an X-ray that was many times larger than the nodule radiologists were searching for. And despite looking right at it, they didn't notice it. I've seen the same phenomenon in clinical case presentations when the client was passed to a new therapist with an existing diagnosis that led the new therapist to miss the gorilla, but in these cases, it was posttraumatic stress disorder, major depression, or obsessive-compulsive disorder. In other words, question everything, especially those things of which you feel certain.

Wisdom from Wilhelm Reich and Sigmund Freud

Memorizing the *DSM* menu of symptoms is no substitute for learning about the functions of the brain, mind, and relationships. Only focusing on current symptoms and diagnoses can result in a catastrophic comprehension of the psychic surface. In other words, you may come up with a correct diagnosis by *DSM* standards while completely missing the client. On the other hand, sometimes a cigar is just a cigar.

Invisible Loyalties

> *There can be grandeur in any degree of submissiveness,*
> *because it springs from loyalty.*
> Simone Weil

Although we experience ourselves as individual beings, we are linked—via our social brains—to our family, friends, culture, and history as far back as our genes can keep track of, which is pretty far. Because humans are fundamentally social creatures, most of our clients' presenting complaints are woven into the fabric of their social lives. The triumphs and failures of our ancestors, both human and prehuman, live within us, shaping our moment-to-moment experience. This is why we have to look beyond symptoms to the person, and beyond the person to the history.

The truth of the matter is that our lives are far too complex to fully comprehend, so we settle on explanations that we can understand and that provide us with some sense of control. People that are certain are certainly wrong—but certainty is seductive. This seductiveness lies in our longing to avoid the anxiety that is triggered by ignorance. Charismatic cult leaders prey on this anxiety and relieve their followers of all doubt. Narcissistic therapists and vulnerable clients can also fall prey to the same regressive dynamic.

One of my favorite quotes from Alcoholics Anonymous is "addicts don't get into relationships, they take hostages." To some degree, this is true of all of us. We get into relationships for a variety of conscious and unconscious reasons, and sometimes we use relationships to play out destructive experiences from our past. The sad truth of many relationships is that we are often unable to salvage them because we have no idea what is happening. Each person feels unloved, misunderstood, and alone and can't understand how the other person doesn't get it. So the therapy office is a crowded place—even when there are only two of you. The client's and therapist's families are sitting inside and around them, activating transference and countertransference reactions and other implicit associations that shape the way we experience and understand one another. While the following case is a dramatic and somewhat unusual example, the dynamics are universal.

Penis Be Gone!

> *Logic is a poor model for cause and effect.*
>
> Gregory Bateson

A striking example of the power of family loyalties was demonstrated by a client I worked with early in my training. John, a young man in his early 20s, became psychotic during boot camp and was sent to a military hospital. His experiences and symptoms were fairly typical for clients diagnosed with schizophrenia except for one thing: during one of his psychotic episodes, he cut his penis off. The treating pharmacologist understood this as a straightforward consequence of his psychosis; his individual psychotherapist interpreted it as an attempt to ward off homosexual impulses, and his nurse thought it was "plain crazy." Everybody had an opinion.

I had no idea what to think and even found focusing on the case extremely difficult. It took me quite a while to get comfortable sitting in the room with him. I kept having intrusive images of him doing the deed, and I experienced twinges of sympathetic pains. The first few sessions were a countertransference festival. Even my supervisors appeared to be having countertransference by proxy. It wasn't until I brought the case to a family therapist that I found a conceptualization I could have confidence in.

In order to treat John, the family therapist told me that the entire immediate family needed to participate—parents, younger brother, and sister—and that he would see them all with me. The thought of seeing the entire family filled me with dread, but at least I would have an ally to help me navigate what I thought would be a tough session. To make matters worse, when one of the supervisors at the hospital got wind of what we were planning, she insisted that the therapy be open to the other trainees for learning purposes. So now I was doing therapy with my most difficult client and his family, with a co-therapist I admired, surrounded by students and staff at the hospital. Going on leave with a stress disability started to look like a good idea.

On the morning of our session, my co-therapist and I sat in an inner circle with five empty seats, surrounded by a larger circle filled with doctors and trainees—including members of the treatment staff whose opinions I described above. As I sat anxiously waiting for John and his family to enter the room, I had to battle with the voices in my head warning me not to make a fool of myself in front of all these people.

Finally, the door opened, and one by one they entered. John entered first, obviously surprised by all of the people in the room. He walked over and took a seat across from me. His mother entered next; the contrast made my head snap back. In walked this very vivacious woman in her early 40s, wearing a skintight t-shirt with the words "Foxy Lady" written in rhinestones across her more than ample bosom. When she saw the crowded room, she had the opposite reaction of John—she lit up as if walking on stage. She flashed her smile as she worked the room and settled down next to her son. As she sat, stretching her pants to the breaking point, she slid her hand down the inside of John's thigh and snuggled into his side. All of our eyes widened as our jaws dropped. We hardly noticed her husband and two other children walk in and sit down. The father sat across from his wife—overweight, depressed, and struggling to move across the room. He fell into his chair and melted in place. The two other children followed suit—carbon copies of their father. We were all speechless. Twenty-year-old men need a very good reason to want their penises gone, and John had one. His loyalty to his father and the family system made his sexual excitement at the hands of his mother untenable. Because no one else in the family had any energy to stand up to her or to set proper boundaries, John's self-mutilation was a solution to a problem that seemed to have no other answer.

Symptoms as expressions of family loyalty don't need to be this extreme. I struggled with going to college because my father gave me many subtle messages not to go before finally telling me that I couldn't. Fortunately for me, I realized that this was an expression of his pain and disappointment from his own childhood that had nothing to do with me. He was very bright but was given the same message by his father. The advantage of growing up in the 1960s was that I had been convinced not to believe what anyone over 30 told me.

I see a similar phenomenon in students who are from backgrounds that don't respect education or that discourage it for women. The weight of these expectations and the invisible loyalties behind them often lead to intense inner conflicts. Bright students don't graduate despite only needing one more semester to get their degree or fail to show up for their final orals to get their doctorate. The symbolic significance of the degree is too much for their inner loyalties to tolerate. Even as adults, the risk of abandonment is too high, so they sabotage their efforts to individuate so as not to threaten their family loyalties.

Many of my clients, especially women in their 50s and beyond, begin to recognize these invisible loyalties and return to school, careers, or other passions with great enthusiasm. It is a great joy for me to help them reach their dreams—a wonderful perk of being a teacher and a therapist.

Spirituality: Healthy and Unhealthy

> *Beware of false knowledge; it is more dangerous than ignorance.*
> George Bernard Shaw

Our clients may also have deep loyalties to their religious beliefs and communities. Unfortunately, psychotherapy and organized religion have not been on the best of terms since Freud referred to religious beliefs as "illusions" and relegated them to Bronze Age superstition. It wasn't until Carl Rogers, a minister's son, and his client-centered therapy that religion and psychotherapy discovered a tense neutral zone. The result has been that students are taught to respect their clients' religious beliefs, which often leads them to consider an interpretation of religious or spiritual beliefs off limits. I believe this is a mistake because religious beliefs and practices can contain important information about nonpresenting problems.

I have witnessed a fair share of what I would describe as pathological spirituality in the press and in my clinical practice. A common example of **pathological spirituality** occurs in clients who are overwhelmed with pathological shame and feel they have no right to any assistance, rest, or happiness. Their full-time role in life is to serve others despite their exhaustion, depression, and rage. These individuals often invoke Buddhist or Christian dogma to justify their selflessness, likening their suffering and sacrifice to those of ascetics and saints.

While martyrdom can be transcendent, it can also serve as a justification for self-hatred that protects clients from the awareness of the deprivation and loss they experienced early in life, an affirmation that both they and their needs are of no importance. Their outward self-sacrifice can hide their secret wish for the good parent to arrive. Children used by narcissistic parents for emotional regulation often grow up to be both generous and angry, magnanimous by day, destructive by night.

Definition: Pathological Spirituality

Broadly defined, pathological spirituality consists of religious beliefs and practices that serve as expressions of unresolved trauma or as psychological defenses. Clear examples are psychopathic cult leaders who use religious dogma to manipulate and abuse others. Slightly less disturbed are the narcissistic televangelists and sex-addled priests who abuse members of their congregation. While these obvious examples hardly need mentioning, and seldom come to therapy, the more common issues in our practices are those who use their religious beliefs to perpetuate maladaptive coping strategies.

On the surface, healthy and unhealthy forms of religion and spirituality often look very much the same. The clues are in whether people's views are open or closed. In other words, are people flexible in their own beliefs and curious about others, or are they rigid, dogmatic, and overly emotional when confronted with alternative perspectives? Do their beliefs encourage them to continue to grow or is there a strong emphasis on obedience and compliance?

In some ways Freud was right about religion, but only half right. For many, religious beliefs have evolved little from Bronze Age superstition and are used to manage anxiety, cope with fear, and keep their demons at bay. Religion is clearly used by many to justify primitive emotions, reinforce prejudices, and avoid the complex issues of living in a pluralistic society. At the same time, others use their religious beliefs to challenge themselves to greater levels of empathy, compassion, and personal accomplishment. This is why a close examination of your clients' spiritual and religious beliefs can potentially provide a great deal of information about their early experiences and inner worlds.

Paranormal Beliefs

I really don't believe in magic.
J. K. Rowling

I have had many clients who frequent psychics or clairvoyants and believe in astral projection, time travel, and telepathic abilities. Although none of them are psychotic, all suffer from symptoms of anxiety and depression and experienced chronic early stress and/or specific traumas. Because of this fairly consistent pattern, I've come to see paranormal beliefs and practices as generally informative about our clients' unremembered past.

Most of the people with these beliefs that I've come to know have made no conscious connection between their strongly held paranormal beliefs and their difficult childhoods. A man in his early 20s, whom I saw for social anxiety, had a firm conviction of his ability to travel through time. He reported to me that he had begun to time travel when he was very young and felt it had saved him from a miserable home life. He had wonderful experiences of visiting famous historical figures, and he had learned a lot about the future that he wasn't at liberty to disclose. During subsequent meetings, he told me that his mother beat him every day from the time he was an infant until his 14th birthday. On his birthday, he asked her to stop; she told him, "Sure!" When he asked her why she beat him every day, her response was, "I thought you liked it." He didn't see his childhood as unusual—it was the only one he had ever had.

Another man in his 30s told me that he possessed the power of transubstantiation—an ability to create matter out of thought. He described an experience when, after a car had cut him off, he concentrated on manifesting a swarm of bees in the offending car. The last thing he remembers of the car was the driver swatting madly at the bees as he drove off the road. Although this man denied being the victim of child abuse, he shared fond memories of playing the bull's-eye game with his father. When I asked him to describe the game, he told me that it included running around the backyard with a bull's-eye t-shirt on while his father used him for target practice with an air rifle. When I asked him if he thought it was dangerous, his response was, "No. I wore goggles." It never occurred to him that being used as a target was an unusual and possibly sadistic father-son pastime.

Finally, a woman in her early 30s with a firm belief in her telepathic abilities shared with me an experience from when she was eight, sitting on a sofa watching television with her four-year-old brother. She heard shots ring out from a drive-by shooting as her baby brother slumped forward—one of the bullets had gone though his tiny head. As an adult, she suffered from generalized anxiety disorder, panic attacks, and agoraphobia. She was inseparable from her mother and sisters. They spoke on the phone hourly and refused to travel without one another. She was convinced that they could read each other's minds and that she could predict when they would call her and what they would say.

All three of these people were in outpatient therapy with various forms of anxiety, did not identify themselves as trauma victims, and were not psychotic. Yet all firmly believed in their paranormal abilities and did not associate these beliefs with their childhood experiences. The symbolic value of escaping abuse by traveling through time, being able to protect oneself through the power of thought, and maintaining psychic connection in the face of overwhelming loss are clear. A psychoanalyst might say that their symbolic value would be more than enough to create and maintain these beliefs—and I might agree. But I think there is more.

Early trauma and chronic stress during childhood have a number of effects on the developing brain—all of which may support the development and maintenance of paranormal beliefs. Neurological attributes associated with trauma, such as smaller hippocampi, larger amygdala, and higher resting levels of cortisol, adrenaline, and endogenous endorphins affect physiological, psychological, and social processing in ways that bring clients to therapy.

Psychotherapy can be especially important for these victims of early stress and trauma because it may be the only context available where they can learn about the distortions of their childhood memories. They can discover how much their minds are committed to beliefs rather than truths, and how early experiences shape our experience of reality. Perhaps most importantly, therapy is a context where clients are exposed to new information that is solely in their best interest, not to meet the needs of those around them.

CHAPTER 4

Using Our Minds to Change Our Brains

Our knowledge can only be finite, while our ignorance must necessarily be infinite.
Karl Popper

A WISE MAN once asked me if I knew the difference between a rat and a human being. "There are many differences," I replied, "whiskers, fur, and tails," all of which were true but left him unimpressed. Here is the story he told me.

If you take a hungry rat and put it on a platform surrounded by five tunnels and you've hidden cheese down the third tunnel, the rat will explore each tunnel until it finds the cheese. Rats have excellent spatial memory, so if you put the same rat in the same place a few days later, it will immediately go down the third tunnel looking for cheese. But, say, after a few days of this, you move the cheese to the fifth tunnel. The rat will continue to go down the third tunnel a number of times looking for the cheese even though it isn't there.

So here is the difference between a rat and a human being. Eventually, the rat will start exploring the other tunnels to find the cheese. Humans, on the other hand, will go down the third tunnel forever because they believe that's where the cheese should be. When we get trapped in patterns that are reinforced by beliefs, theories, and "good ideas," it is clear that our **brains** are not serving us and that our **minds** are not our friends. We often see this in our clients and ourselves as we continue to employ the same unsuccessful strategies in our lives with continued negative results. This is all the more impactful when it is clear that, in other areas of life, we may be very successful. We may even be the one others come to for advice and guidance. The same phenomenon occurs when therapists continue to employ failing strategies and techniques with a client and attribute our lack of progress to our clients' resistance.

One way to conceptualize emotional distress is to continue doing the same thing, in the same way, hoping for different results. In other words, people keep going down the third tunnel, find no cheese, and try it again. The cheese might be love, or success at work, or simply finding peace of mind. But no matter how much they employ the same strategy, they come up empty handed until they accept the fact that they may benefit from a new strategy.

Definition: Mind and Brain

Our brains consist of the wetware of our nervous system —the millions of cells that comprise the neural networks traveling throughout our bodies. Our minds emerge from our nervous systems, consisting of memory, consciousness, and self-awareness. The ways our brains are shaped play a large bottom-up role in shaping our minds, while our minds are capable of changing our brains through conscious changes in our thoughts, actions, and emotions.

The good news about rats is that they are pragmatic, flexible, and unburdened by becoming attached to unsuccessful strategies. While I'd rather be a human than a rat, sometimes we have to think more like a rat to succeed. There is an array of cognitive-based therapies that try to utilize our rat brains by helping us to root out and question dysfunctional or irrational beliefs.

When Your Mind Is Not Your Friend

> *Where ignorance is our master, there is no possibility of real peace.*
> Dalai Lama

Human brains are capable of creating everything from cheeseburgers to impressionism. Because of our accomplishments, especially in comparison to other animals, we like to think of ourselves as quite superior. Add to this our technological accomplishments, including computers, space flight, and microsurgery, and we are altogether smug about having reached some evolutionary apex. However, our focus on technical accomplishments and mastery over other animals tends to obscure how poorly we understand and control our own thoughts, behaviors, and emotions.

Our brains and minds are full of information and churn out thoughts and feelings a mile a minute; some good, some not so good, some just terrible. Unfortunately, it is often hard for us to tell the difference. The front page of any major newspaper pays testimony to how unsophisticated humans are in vitally important matters. Beneath a thin veneer of civility, we remain primitive animals driven by overheated emotion, distorted thinking, and unconscious egocentrism. These are not character flaws or psychiatric disorders, but natural consequences of our evolutionary histories.

A good example is depression, which can lead our brains around like a dog on a leash. A change in biochemistry that causes us to slip into depression makes a life that looked fine yesterday look like a nightmare today. The only thing that may have changed is your serotonin level. So yesterday you were making plans for winter vacation, and today you are thinking of ways to kill yourself so that you don't leave too much of a mess. You may not even remember how good your life was yesterday.

While medication can do wonders for many of us who struggle with depression, we still have to learn to be aware of our minds and to manage them with care, which allows us to quickly realize, "Oh, I'm thinking about jumping out of the window. My brain chemistry must have shifted. I better be really good to myself today, not make any important decisions, and not take anything my mind suggests too seriously—today, my mind is not my friend." A therapist can assist clients with recognizing mood states that negatively skew their perception of reality and help them to develop strategies to better manage their off days.

Eating Into Unconsciousness

> *Being unconscious is the ultimate disability.*
> Jessa Gamble

Years ago, I was telling my therapist that I wished I could get in better shape but that despite all my efforts, I always felt a few days away from getting there. "If only I could eat better," I told her. In good therapeutic form, she replied, "Tell me more." I told her that I exercised almost every day, ate a lot of healthy produce, and watched my weight. On most days, I ate well all day until the evening. At some point during the evening, I would shift into a state of mind where I would eat lots of sweets and junk food. I suppose you could call it binge eating, but because I was in such good shape and not overweight, I never labeled it that way. But it was clear that the number and kind of calories I was eating most evenings was not good.

The more I spoke of my evening binges, the more I became aware of how automatic and unconscious the behavior was and how out of control I felt about it. As the session ended, she suggested that I think about it more, which I promptly forgot until a few days later. One morning, as I lay in bed in between sleep and waking, a memory that felt like a daydream began to play in my mind.

I was a young boy, perhaps seven or eight, walking into the kitchen where my grandmother was cleaning up. I was sad about something or other, and instead of responding to my words or feelings, she gradually turned to the right and opened the refrigerator. She reached into the freezer and pulled out a half-gallon box of ice cream. As she turned back in my direction, she pulled off the paper zippers, grabbed a spoon, and pushed it into the ice cream. I put out my arms, and she placed the large box of ice cream in my hands. As I walked away, she draped a dishcloth over my shoulders. I lay down on the sofa with the ice cream on my chest, eating spoonful after spoonful of the delicious stuff until I entered a sugar-induced stupor.

An important thing to know about my family is that the direct expression of negative feelings was rare, and discussions about emotions were nonexistent. There was a special injunction against sadness, something I only realized later in life. There had been enough tragedy, loss, and heartbreak already, and I, as the first child of a new generation, was to be saved from sadness. This meant that expressing sadness needed to be staved off at all costs. Food was a way to distance us from emotions, especially negative ones. Unfortunately, it left me without a language with which to understand the painful aspects of my inner world.

In addition to opening up a valuable avenue in my therapy, I also learned about a technique used in Alcoholics Anonymous for increasing self-awareness called HALT. When you feel like having a drink, say the word "HALT," and ask yourself whether you are hungry, angry, lonely, or tired. The idea is that if you are going for a drink, there is probably some emotion triggering the need for it. Of course, there can be other emotions, but they wouldn't spell HALT, which is quite useful.

HALT not only reminds you to not drink (or eat in my case) but also to be self-reflective and to engage in a caring relationship with yourself. You are doing what a good parent should do, saying, "I can see something is wrong; tell me what you are experiencing." The added awareness interrupts a chain of internal cause-and-effect relationships that provide you with the opportunity to reflect, reconsider, and redirect. This is where well-established and mature relationships with your inner world come in handy.

Using the HALT technique is a way to use your mind to change your brain. Asking yourself what you are feeling instead of engaging in reflexive behavior allows your mind to reconnect with your primitive brain. In a sense, you are giving yourself what you needed as a child—to be seen, to feel felt, and articulate your experiences in a healthy way. This internal reparenting will eventually integrate neural circuitry that will allow you to replace symptoms with functional adaptations. In my case, it meant taking better care of myself, investing more in relationships, and being willing to confront pain.

Bearing Witness

> *All truths are easy to understand once they are discovered.*
> Galileo Galilei

Because we are profoundly social creatures that share in a group mind, reality is in large part a social construction. Things become more real, more solid when we know they are being seen by others. Children demonstrate this in a very straightforward way when they repeatedly implore their parents, "Watch this, watch this!" as they do a cartwheel or balance a box on their heads. Having a witness activates social brain systems, which makes most of us aware of how we look to others and provides a more objective perspective to our singular egocentric view.

Fear and terror often lead us to disconnect from shared experience. I have had clients from Baghdad, Beirut, and London, separated by culture, language, and generations, but sharing the experience of having been in buildings that were destroyed by bombs. They all described the same experience—hearing the whistling growing louder, the explosion, the violent movements, the long periods of dead silence, struggling to breathe through the clouds of dust, and the search for the bodies of loved ones.

Another client, fleeing on foot from Eastern Europe to escape the Nazis, was crossing a field with his older brother. A fighter plane dropped a bomb that landed within feet of where they had taken cover. They stared at the bomb, waiting for it to explode, frozen, not knowing what to do. A young woman I worked with was driven to the desert by her sadistic husband and forced to dig her own grave as he sat and sharpened his knife. These are all experiences that terrify us to the point where we go into shock, lose our words, and become fragmented. The trauma gets locked within us and becomes the soundtrack of our inner emotional lives.

The value of a witness to horror can never be overestimated. Someone who is willing to go with us to the ground zero of our pain helps us to be able to sit with it ourselves. Having to communicate our story to another encourages us to articulate an experience that may only be a series of images, bodily sensations, and emotions. Having to make our experiences comprehensible to another person allows us to grasp them in a clearer and more empowering way. Telling the story also provides us with the opportunity to see the reaction of the other, which helps us to grasp the emotional meaning of our experiences. In addition, telling the story to others provides us with a new memory of the story that now includes a witness, making it a public experience. Once we have an articulated story, we have the ability to edit it—something that doesn't exist when an experience is composed of images and emotions existing out of time.

The ability to heal psychic pain by telling our story to others has been shaped into our brains over a hundred thousand years, long before therapy came along, and now reframed as a professional intervention. When young therapists hear these stories, they feel that they have to do something with the information in order to earn their keep. Over time, we come to more deeply appreciate the fact that simply bearing witness is an important part of our job. Sometimes the best thing to do is to do nothing but listen, which is exactly what is needed.

Expanding Self-Awareness

Meditation is participatory observation.
Buddha

Like putting feelings into words, learning to look inward and becoming self-aware is something that has to be learned. In exploring our inner worlds, we come to learn that our minds use language in different ways. In fact, through self-reflection, most of us become aware that we seem to shift among different perspectives, emotional states, and types of inner self-talk. At least three levels of language processing arise during different states of mind: a reflexive social language, an internal dialogue, and a language of self-reflection.

Reflexive social language (RSL) is a stream of words that appears to exist in the service of maintaining ongoing social connection. Primarily a function of the brain's left hemisphere, RSL mirrors activity within the interpersonal world and is designed to facilitate social interactions. Verbal reflexes, clichés, and overlearned reactions in social situations provide a meaningful web of connection with those around us. The best example is the obligatory "How are you? Fine; how are you? Fine. See you later." Most of us also experience this level of language whenever we automatically say something positive to avoid conflict or when we tell people we are "fine" regardless of what's troubling us. The natural clichés of RSL are as automatic to us as walking and breathing, serving the same purpose in human groups as grooming and play do in other primates.

In fact, they seem to be more like motor reflexes than real expressions of our thoughts or feelings.

In addition to RSL, we are also aware of the conversations that go on inside our heads. This internal dialogue is a private language that often differs in content and tone from what we typically express to others. While RSL is driven by social cooperation, internal dialogue is experienced as a single voice or a conversation, usually with a negative emotional tone. Internal language may have evolved on a separate track from social language to allow for private thought. This automatic, sometimes compulsive flow of thoughts is most often driven by fear, doubt, and shame. "Did I lock the back door? I'm so stupid! Do I look fat in these pants?"

This voice is likely driven by the right hemisphere, as it is agrammatical and usually negative in tone. Unfortunately, it is also a key way that right-hemisphere processing contributes to conscious awareness. It is the inner voice of our shadow that undermines our confidence and the critical voice that gossips about others. RSL and internal dialogue are both reflexive and habitual, and they serve to maintain preexisting attitudes, behaviors, and feelings. RSL is an expression of how we have been taught to interact with other people; our internal language reflects how we have learned to feel about ourselves, our attachments, and our social status. So while RSL keeps us in line with the group, internal dialogue keeps us on the track that our parents placed us on at the beginning of our lives.

While most of our time is spent bouncing back and forth between RSL and internal dialogue, every once in awhile we attain a state of mind that allows us to observe both our RSL and internal dialogue. It is as if we find an internal quiet from which to reflect apart from the compulsive flow of words, thoughts, and actions. This third level, self-reflective language, is a vehicle of thoughtful consideration. It employs our executive functions and imagination to attain an objective view of our experience. Guiding our clients to become aware of these different kinds of internal languages and states of mind supports an expansion of self-awareness, emotional regulation, and learning.

Learning that we are more than the voices that haunt us can provide hope and serve as a means of changing our lives. As the language of self-awareness is expanded and reinforced, we learn that we are capable of choosing whether or not to follow the expectations of others and the mandates of our childhoods and cultures. Thus, much of our suffering can be traced back to our stream of thoughts, the voices in our heads, and the stories we tell about ourselves.

What Would Buddha Do?

> *Do not dwell in the past, do not dream of the future,*
> *concentrate the mind on the present moment.*
> Buddha

While Buddhism contains many valuable life lessons, one of the most important is the difference between pain and suffering. Pain is woven into nature and is an inevitable part of life. To desire results in disappointment; to love means you will experience loss, and to be born naturally leads to aging and death. By contrast, suffering is what our minds make of these experiences when they are not at hand. Suffering is the anguish we experience from worry about not getting the things we need or from losing the things that we have. It is the anticipatory anxiety and catastrophic thinking we connect with not wearing the right jeans, failing to getting straight As, or not getting married and having a baby according to schedule. Suffering is what our minds create to make us dissatisfied and crazy, no matter how much we have.

Driven by extreme emotions and errant biochemical states, our minds appear to have a predilection for moving from the rational to the irrational. When fear evokes the amygdala's primitive executive powers, anticipatory anxiety moves toward catastrophic thinking and turns worst-case scenarios into the most likely outcome. Shades of gray become black-and-white choices leading to all-or-nothing outcomes with life-and-death consequences. Visibility will lead to being exposed as a fraud, banishment from the tribe, and even stoning. Reflect for a moment on an old fable of a man facing death.

The Strawberry and the Tigers

A man traveling across a field encountered a tiger. He fled, the tiger after him. Coming to a precipice, he caught hold of the root of a wild vine and swung himself down over the edge. The tiger sniffed at him from above. Trembling, the man looked down to where, far below, another tiger was waiting to eat him. Only the vine sustained him. Two mice, one white and one black, little by little started to gnaw away the vine. The man saw a luscious strawberry near him. Grasping the vine with one hand, he plucked the strawberry with the other. How sweet it tasted!

While most of us would never claim to have the equanimity of the man in this fable, the message is clear. Although we all hang from the same vine, our minds focus on the tigers and miss the strawberries—this is why we suffer. Buddha's goal, enlightenment, was to end suffering by extinguishing desire, passion, and self.

Most clients don't come to therapy to become enlightened, but most do need to become less symptomatic, to get out of their own way, and to become more engaged in life—to be free to love and work. A reasonable goal. Although the goal of therapy is not to become enlightened, some of the strategies are similar to Buddhist practices. In fact, you may have already spotted some of the similarities between the Buddhist notion of pain and suffering and some things you already know about Rational Emotive Behavior Therapy. Ellis noticed these tendencies of the mind and developed strategies to use rational thinking to battle our irrational ones.

Being Mindful

> *Ignorance is always afraid of change.*
> Jawaharlal Nehru

Being mindful involves remembering that we have a mind, which is not as easy as it sounds. While our bowels and bladders remind us of their existence, our minds are silent and unpresuming, preferring to go unnoticed. There is no reflex to orient us to the mind's existence, no pressure exerted or guilt employed if we ignore it. Thus, being mindful involves effort and discipline. This is why many people go through life without realizing that they have a mind.

If and when we do manage to remember that we have a

mind, then what? What do I do with this mind I've discovered? One of the first things you may notice when you become aware of your mind is that it keeps generating thoughts whether you want it to or not. There may be a momentary interruption in the flow when you take your first look, but soon enough, it goes back to its incessant stream of thoughts and images. But what you now have is the ability to observe the process playing across a kind of inner stage. The next thing you realize is that this stream of thought goes on without conscious effort or intention. It doesn't even need you to identify with it. So all of this stuff that your mind is generating is coming from inside of you, but it isn't all of you. After all, who is paying attention to the stream of consciousness? That's you, too.

By realizing you are not just a continuous stream of thoughts, images, and behaviors, you can make some choices that you couldn't make before. You can take your mind on a tour around the inside of your body to see and feel tension and pain in this place or that. It is surprising to discover how much tension we hold in certain places and how completely unaware of it we can be. On the other hand, paying close attention to a pleasing smell, focusing your consciousness, or moving to a deep muscle stretch can be very soothing.

Another thing you can do is to take a trip into the minds of other people. Once you establish some individuation from your own stream of consciousness, you can imagine what the world looks like from the perspective of others. Even more valuable, you can imagine how they experience you and even their side of a disagreement or difference of opinion. Mindfulness offers you the opportunity to consider how someone else might be right, an extremely valuable interpersonal tool. Since this way of thinking isn't reflexive for us, perhaps natural selection doesn't think it is too important to have mindful awareness. In fact, some evolutionary theorists think that self-awareness may actually be detrimental to survival because it slows down our response to potentially dangerous situations or makes us doubt ourselves and hesitate when we need to act.

Let's assume that the fears of evolutionary biologists are based on animals in natural settings, not modern humans in technologically advanced cultures. Given our present environment and the dense matrix of social connections in which we live, thinking before we act may become increasingly important for human survival. One of the benefits of mindfulness is creating the time to think between impulse and action. And a benefit of exploring our bodies for pain and tension is that stressors sometimes take physical form, which provides insight into what is going on in our brains and unconscious minds.

Becoming the CEO of Your Self

Peace comes from within.
Buddha

A client I'll call Shaun sat across from me looking exasperated and hopeless. "Why am I haunted by these voices? My life is great. I've made it, so why can't I just enjoy it? When the voices aren't criticizing me, they are second guessing everything I do." I knew Shaun well; I also knew that these voices weren't a sign of psychosis. "I know. They suck, don't they?" I replied. "You hear them too?" he asked. I responded, "Absolutely, never remember a time without them." "Well, where do they come from, and where do I go for an exorcism?" he asked. I smiled and said, "I have a theory.

"The human brain has had a long and complex evolutionary history, and I believe that these voices are a kind of archae-ological artifact. Each of us has two brains, one on the left and one on the right. Long ago, primates had brains that were largely the same on both sides, but as our brains became larger and more complicated, they began to specialize in different skills and abilities. The right hemisphere is in control of very high and very low levels of emotion (terror and shame) and is likely a model for what both hemispheres were once like. It also has an early developmental spurt in the first 18 months of life and connects with caretakers for the purposes of attach-ment, emotional regulation, and a sense of self.

"The left hemisphere veered off from this path, specializ-ing in later-evolving abilities such as language, rational thought, and other qualities that probably led to our ability to have self-awareness. The left hemisphere is largely in control during the day, with the right hemisphere feeding it informa-tion from the background. Both hemispheres have language; the left hemisphere has the language we use to think through problems and to communicate with others. The right has a language that is primitive, nonsyntactic, and usually fearful and negative in tone. It is the worrier and the critic. These voices are part of the right hemisphere's input into conscious experience."

"Well, that does suck!" Shaun said. "But why are they so negative?"

"Well, we know that the right hemisphere is biased toward negativity, and people with more activation in the right than the left prefrontal cortex tend to be depressive. This was prob-ably shaped because being negative and suspicious most likely correlated with survival in earlier environments. The right hemisphere is completely wrapped up in survival, the way both of our hemispheres once were. The best guess I have is that the voices in our heads are the right-hemisphere remnants of voices of parents and tribal leaders that kept us coordinated with the group and behaving in ways that kept the group safe. Freud called this the **superego**.

Definition: Superego

In order for animals to become social beings, a balance must be struck between the needs of the individual, others, and the group as a whole. Freud referred to the internalization of the expectations and demands of society as the superego.

"Remember that the purpose of the brain is to enhance survival through the prediction and control of future outcomes. More specifically, the right hemisphere, biased toward anxiety and shame, wants us to always worry about whether we are acceptable to others, if we are going to get fired, and is always anticipating anxiety and shame. Concern about the future and being accepted by the group appear to have been woven into our genes, brains, and minds. Some of us have especially harsh and critical voices that never let up. This may be because we had critical parents, have a bias toward depression, or lack self-confidence and feel ashamed of who we are.

"Because these voices seem to come from deep inside of us, we forget that they are memories, and we come to identify them as who we really are. A central aspect of taking control of our lives is to understand the voices as memory programming errors and learn how to interpret, manage, and mitigate their negative effects. I'm not sure they ever go away. We may even need them in other instances when their advice is accurate and actually helpful. But we all need to learn which of these voices are counterproductive and to tell them to get lost. This is one way that understanding how your brain evolved and developed can turn your mind into your friend."

I'm sure that Shaun had heard the message of not paying attention to these thoughts many times before. Whether or not the explanation I presented to him is correct, it captured his attention and imagination. He was able to label these voices as something other than the "truth" about himself. This scientific narrative created a way for him to objectify his enemy—these shaming and critical right-hemisphere voices—and to develop strategies to fight them. This neuroscientific explanation and the explanation of irrational thoughts in Cognitive-Behavioral Therapy are not the same. I'm not telling Shaun that he is being irrational. I am saying that the voices in his head need to be separated from his self-identity. He now has an enemy to tackle.

CHAPTER 5

Those Things We Don't Remember Yet Never Forget

The past is never dead. It's not even the past.
William Faulkner

FREUD BELIEVED THAT a fundamental goal of therapy is to make the unconscious conscious. I would phrase it a slightly different way. The goal of therapy is to expand conscious awareness and to increase the integration of the various neural networks dedicated to unconscious and conscious memory.

Change in psychotherapy is all about memory: the exploration of past memory, the impact of the past on the present, and the ability to modify what is stored in memory to affect changes in thoughts, feelings, and behaviors. This makes understanding the evolution, development, and functioning of our various memory systems crucial to psychotherapists. It is also very helpful in explaining some of the paradoxes and confusion clients experience based on the ways their brains process information.

The unconscious networks of memory shape our perception and understanding of the world microseconds before we become aware of our perceptions. Through these mechanisms, our past experiences create our expectations for the future. Implicit, unconscious memories, created in dysfunctional situations years before, can repeatedly lead us to re-create unsuccessful but familiar patterns of thought, emotion, and behavior. Most psychological disorders cause anxiety and trigger the secretion of cortisol, which damages the hippocampus and negatively impacts memory functions, reality testing, and emotional regulation. Depression, for example, results in a negative bias in the recollection and interpretation of memory. It also leads us to selectively scan the environment in ways that reinforce negative perceptions.

The Complexity of Memory

Gratitude is when memory is stored in the heart and not in the mind.
Lionel Hampton

Although we tend to think of memory only as the conscious recall of information, research, clinical practice, and everyday life support the existence of many systems of memory. Each system has its own domains of learning, neural architecture, and developmental timetable. The two broadest categories of memory are explicit and implicit.

Explicit memory describes conscious learning and memory, including semantic, sensory, and motor forms. These systems provide for conscious, contextualized memory that becomes more consistent and stable as we develop. These memory systems allow us to recite the alphabet, recognize the smell of coconut, and play tennis. Some of these memory abilities remain just beneath the level of consciousness until we turn our attention to them. **Implicit memory** is reflected in unconscious patterns of learning that are largely inaccessible to conscious awareness. This category extends from repressed traumatic memories, to riding a bicycle, to getting queasy when we smell food that once made us sick. Explicit memory is the tip of our experiential iceberg; implicit memory is the vast infrastructure below the surface.

Definition: Implicit and Explicit Memory

Implicit Memory	*Explicit Memory*
Early developing, subcortical bias	Later developing, cortical bias
Right-hemisphere bias	Left-hemisphere bias
Amygdala centered, orbital and medial prefrontal cortex (OMPFC)	Hippocampal, dorsal lateral prefrontal cortex
Context free, no source attribution	Contextualized, known memory source

Implicit Social Memory	*Explicit Social Memory*
Attachment schema	Identity and social information
Transference	Narratives
Superego	Autobiographical descriptions
Background affect	Social rules, norms, expectations

Because of the order in which they develop, implicit and explicit memory are referred to as early and late memory. Systems of implicit memory come online even before birth, as demonstrated in the newborn's recognition of her mother's voice. These early-forming neural networks depend on the more primitive brain structures such as the amygdala, thalamus, and middle portions of the frontal cortex. The development of conscious memory parallels the maturation of the hippocampus and higher cortical structures over the first decades of life. The absence of explicit memories from early life likely results from this maturational delay. Thus, we learn how to walk and talk, whether the world is safe or dangerous, and how to attach to others in the absence of explicit memory. These vital early lessons are known even though we don't remember learning them.

For most of us, words and visual images are the keys to conscious memory. Different types of semantic memory include episodic, narrative, and autobiographical, which can all be organized sequentially. Autobiographical memory combines episodic, semantic, and emotional memory with a first-person perspective. This form of memory is especially important for the formation and maintenance of emotional regulation, self-identity, and the transmission of culture. It is also a central lever in psychotherapy. Psychotherapy often involves the integration and retrieval of unconscious emotional and somatic memories stored in subcortical and right-hemisphere structures with conscious memories primarily stored in the left hemisphere.

Amygdala Versus Hippocampus

> *It's surprising how much memory is built around things that*
> *go unnoticed at the time.*
>
> Barbara Kingsolver

The amygdala, our primitive executive brain, is central to processing experience during early life. It is fully developed by the eighth month of gestation; even before birth, we are capable of experiencing intense physiological states of fear. During the first few years of life we are dependent on caretakers for external modulation of the amygdala until we are able to self-regulate. Despite the amygdala's later eclipse by the cortex as a general executive center during waking hours, it retains its role as a central hub of social and emotional processing throughout life. Thus, good parents, therapists, and coaches learn to be amygdala whisperers in order to soothe those in their care.

The amygdala functions as an organ of appraisal for danger, safety, and familiarity in approach-avoidance situations. It assists in connecting emotional value to external objects based on instincts and learning history; it then translates these appraisals into bodily states. The amygdala's direct neural connectivity with the hypothalamus and many brain stem nuclei allows it to trigger rapid survival responses. Important for psychotherapy is the fact that it plays a behind-the-scene role in assessing the social environment for danger. In building a therapeutic alliance, we are attempting to downregulate amygdala activation. When the amygdala does become activated and our clients become afraid, we can gain valuable information about how their amygdala have been programmed.

Whereas the amygdala has a central role in the emotional

and somatic organization of experience, the hippocampus is vital for conscious, logical, and cooperative social functioning. The hippocampus is not only essential for expert learning, it also participates in our ability to compare different memories and make inferences from previous learning in new situations. The hippocampus is noted for its late maturation, with the myelination of cortical-hippocampal circuits continuing into adulthood. The late development of the hippocampus results in a prolonged sensitivity to developmental disruption and traumatic insult.

We can immediately see the relevance of the interacting amygdala and hippocampal memory systems to our work in psychotherapy. The amygdala memory system retains early and traumatic memories that, if activated, will impact us by activating fear responses. For example, early abandonment terror stored in implicit memory systems makes the patient with borderline personality disorder see abandonment where little or none exists because for humans and other young primates, abandonment means death.

Therapy with this patient would utilize the hippocampal-cortical systems to test the reality of these amygdala-triggered cues for abandonment in order to inhibit inappropriate reactions. This reality testing, a core component of Dialectical Behavior Therapy (DBT), helps us distinguish real abandonment from innocent triggers, such as someone showing up a few minutes late for an appointment, and inhibit the life-and-death emotional reactions preserved from childhood. The catastrophic reaction of borderline patients to abandonment is a result of the fact that it is experienced, as it is for all of us in our earliest days, as a threat to survival.

Memories from early and traumatic experiences, such as

abandonment, reside in amygdala-driven memory networks. Flashbacks are excellent examples of amygdala-based memories that are inadequately modulated by cortical executive systems. Because of how they are wired, PTSD victims' flashbacks are powerful and multisensory, often triggered by stress, and are experienced as if they are occurring in the present. These flashbacks also have the characteristic of being repetitive, suggesting that they are not subject to the assimilating and contextualizing properties of the cortex.

The amygdala strives to generalize, while the hippocampus tries to discriminate. In other words, the amygdala will make us jump at the sight of a spider, while the hippocampus will soon allow us to remember that this particular spider is not poisonous, so there's no need to flee. Given the reciprocal nature of amygdala and hippocampal circuits, impairment of the hippocampus should lead to an increased influence of the amygdala in directing memory, emotion, and behavior. This imbalance toward the amygdala also disrupts affect regulation. For example, depressed patients are overwhelmed by their negative feelings and unable to engage in adequate reality testing. Dysregulation of hippocampal-amygdala circuits are likely involved in both depressive symptomatology and disturbed reality testing.

The Intrusion of Implicit Memory Into Conscious Awareness

> *Dreaming ties all mankind together.*
> Jack Kerouac

Although implicit memories are actively kept out of conscious awareness, they influence our conscious experiences and behaviors. Clients often come to therapy when their implicit memory systems impact their lives in negative ways that impede their abilities to love and work. One of the many ways in which implicit memory impacts our day-to-day lives is through our attachment schema. Attachment schema guide and shape relationships throughout life. Given that so many clients come to therapy with relationship difficulties, this implicit memory system may be one of the most important to understand and explore. The same networks of social memory give rise to the phenomenon of transference, a process that brings these early unconscious memories into the consulting room to be played out between client and therapist. Enactments in psychotherapy, involving the interplay between unconscious elements within the patient and the therapist, also activate these implicit memories. Enactments are, in essence, the implicit memory systems of both client and therapist engaging in ways of interacting, of which neither is fully aware.

We have all had our buttons pushed by someone; many of these buttons are the emotional traces of personal experiences stored in implicit memory. Overreacting to something implies that the difference between an appropriate reaction and how we actually react is attributable to a sensitivity based on past experience. The most common distortions are related to shame, a primary physiological state that develops during our first year. Individuals with core shame can find criticism, rejection, and abandonment in nearly every interaction, which can result in a life of chronic anxiety, perfectionism, exhaustion, and depression.

Silence may be golden, but in therapy it is an ambiguous stimulus that can evoke a variety of implicit memories. Often, our clients reaction to silence during sessions can teach us about their emotional history. During periods of silence, many clients assume that the therapist is thinking critical thoughts about them, imagining that the therapist thinks they are boring, stupid, a waste of time, or a bad client. These feelings usually mirror those from problematic relationships with one or both parents. Furthermore, these feelings are deep seated and tenacious. On the other hand, some clients find silence to be a form of acceptance and a relief from the pressures of active interactions. These stark differences in clients' reactions to the same experience are convincing evidence of the workings of implicit memory and their effects on conscious experience.

A similar phenomenon occurs in individuals who become uncomfortable when they try to relax without any distractions. The emotions, images, and thoughts that emerge in the absence of distraction may hold clues to the aftereffects of early learning. Defenses against these negative feelings often require the victim to engage in constant action to keep from becoming frightened or overwhelmed, a process sometimes called a manic defense. It often takes many years to make implicit memories conscious so that we can examine and modify them.

Head-Stuck Dreams

> Reality is never as bad as a nightmare, as the mental tortures
> we inflict on ourselves.
> Sammy Davis, Jr.

Many of my clients have discovered yoga and meditation as helpful adjuncts to psychotherapy. In addition to helping them become more aware of how their minds process information, they often report a deeper sense of their bodily reactions that they can use to become more aware of their emotions. These are good things that can be supportive of the therapeutic process. The combination of tuning out distractions and turning inward can also lead to the release of implicit memories that are inhibited under normal circumstances. I experienced a powerful example of this early in my training.

As part of a meditation training program, I spent long periods sitting in a chair being led through what were called body processes. These processes were forms of guided imagery in which the leader encouraged us to "find a space" in various parts of our bodies. The idea was to become more aware of our bodies, including the tension held in different muscle groups, and to be more receptive to whatever thoughts, feelings, and memories emerged.

As I sat through these meditation exercises, I was often bored and struggled to keep my mind focused on the task. As the hours went by, my mind wandered, and my stomach and bladder seemed to have control of my thoughts. Enlightenment was nowhere on the horizon. Somewhere in the midst of my random thoughts, I began to have a strong physical sensation. My entire body felt as if I was being squeezed into a ball by the contractions of my stomach muscles. I have no idea what caused this to happen, but I became transfixed by what was happening to my body. I began to wonder if I was having a heart attack, but was so fascinated that it didn't occur to me to call out for help.

As these contractions continued, I could no longer stay on my chair, and I slowly rolled onto the carpet. As I lay next to my chair, I became aware that my body was completely covered with sweat although I had been cool only moments earlier. At this point my mind offered me a visual image. I could see myself in King Kong's hand being squeezed into a ball. The pressure was intense, and for a moment I imagined I was being carried up a tall building.

I could still hear the voice of the group leader instructing us to find a place in various parts of our bodies. His voice sounded far away, and it was hard to believe that a crowd hadn't gathered around me. The pressure and the heat were intense and seemed to go on for quite some time. Then, out of nowhere came a sharp pain deep in the muscles of my left jaw. It felt as if I were being cut with a knife from my chin upward toward my left ear. I reflexively pulled both hands to my face. I lay there fascinated and frightened. It was like having a dream while being awake.

After another period of time, I began to feel the pressure around my feet and ankles ease with a simultaneous cooling. The next change was a similar experience on my lower legs and up to my thighs. It felt like whatever was holding me was slowly letting go, as if King Kong's fingers were releasing one at a time. This continued up through my torso, but I noticed the pace slowed a bit when it reached my shoulders. Finally, and all at once, the pressure on my shoulders and head was released, and I lay there cool, relaxed, and exhausted. My awareness slowly returned to the room. The voice of the leader was still directing the body meditation, and I had no idea how long I had been captivated by this experience.

My growing self-consciousness led me to get up onto my chair. It was approximately four in the afternoon. There were still many hours and many different aspects of the training to go. We weren't let out of the room until three the next morning and were also due back in six hours. Despite the power of this experience, the distractions and my lack of understanding led me to forget it had even happened.

More than a month later, I was sitting with my mother and remembered the experience, and I described it to her as you have just read it. As I went through my explanation, her eyes widened, and she was unusually attentive. Stunned, she launched into a description of my birth, which included a long and difficult labor, a breach birth with instruments that cut the left side of my face, and two weeks in intensive care. When she was done, she guided me to the bathroom and turned my head to the side, revealing a faint scar on my left cheek (of which I was unaware) where I had felt the pain during the meditation.

At the time, although it was an interesting coincidence, I did not believe that we were capable of remembering our births. I was 23 years old and fancied myself a bit of a junior scientist. My mother had her share of superstitions and even believed that there might be something to astrology. It was an open-and-shut case. I didn't know what had happened, but I was sure that it wasn't a birth experience. It did feel like my body was possessed by some kind of force, but it certainly couldn't have been a memory from a time before I remembered anything. I still believed that memory was conscious and monolithic. Once again, this experience passed from my thoughts.

Two months later, I was preparing for bed when a powerful thought struck me. It had been several months since the last time I had a dream where my head got stuck. As far back as I could remember, I had recurring nightmares of getting my head stuck three or four times a week. There was a vast range of scenarios: I would be swimming under the ice gasping for air, and I would spot a hole in the ice and swim toward it. It would be too small for my head and I would feel like I was going to drown, panic, and then wake up. I would be walking down a staircase in an office building and the stairs would narrow, as in an Escher painting, to an opening that would be too small for my head. If I had kept journals throughout my childhood, I could have recorded hundreds of different situations resulting in the same experience.

In these dreams, my thought was always the same: if I could only get my head through, the rest of my body would follow. Even in the dreams the thought would confuse me because I knew that my shoulders were much larger than my head. In these dreams, despite my knowledge of the realities of my physical body, I knew that my head was the obstacle and that my torso would not present a problem. This was a physical reality that was true at birth, but certainly not in adulthood.

As I sat there astounded by the fact that these dreams had stopped, I also became aware that I had never told anyone about them. In fact, they were such a normal part of my life that I just took them for granted. Now that they were gone, I felt simultaneously relieved, sad, and confused. I strained to remember when I had had the last dream. It finally dawned on me that it had been before the meditation training. I finally made the connection.

I was full of questions. Had I "reexperienced" my birth? Did being with my mother trigger the memory of the experience in meditation class? Had decades of repetitive dreams resulted from the trauma of my birth? The truth is, I don't know the answers to any of these questions. But the power of this experience combined with the discontinuing of the dreams suggests a number of possibilities. One is that memories can be repressed or represented symbolically in other ways. Another is that we have multiple memory systems that can become dissociated and later reintegrated.

If the story described above is related to my birth, our bodies may have fairly complex memories resulting from the earliest experiences of fear. In my case, there were physical sensations of pressure, temperature, and pain linked with a sense of danger and panic. And just as important is that these primitive memories become expressed symbolically in dreams and in symptoms such as anxiety or depression during waking hours. The value of this experience has been to convince me of the power of nonconscious memory and its impact on cognitive, emotional, and social development. By definition, clients will never tell you what is stored in their implicit memory. Our job is to listen between the lines, go beyond the information given, and look carefully at the missing parts of a client's narrative. The clues to implicit memory are in the dark places.

The Plasticity of Memory

> *The older I get, the better I was.*
> Van Dyke Parks

Research into false memory has highlighted many shortcomings in the knowledge of therapists. Highly publicized legal cases have shone a bright light on clinicians' contribution to the co-construction of false memories. Most therapists are now aware of the vulnerability of conscious memory to suggestion, distortion, and fabrication from both client and therapist. Research has demonstrated that memory can be implanted in experimental situations where the subject soon becomes certain that the false memories have actually occurred. A therapist's belief that her client has been abused may influence that patient to unconsciously fabricate a memory that he or she comes to believe as true. This process is a clear demonstration of both the malleability of memory and the power of co-constructed narrative in shaping experience.

The malleability of memory is an observable manifestation of the plasticity of these neural systems. Revisiting and evaluating childhood experiences from an adult perspective often leads to rewriting history in a creative and positive way. The introduction of new information or scenarios to past experiences can alter the nature of memories and modify affective reactions. The good news here is that painful memories can be altered by subsequent experiences. This is a lot of what we do in psychotherapy and part of the answer to the question of why therapy works.

PART TWO
The Social Brain
Embodied and Embedded

CHAPTER 6

The Social Brain and Failure to Thrive

We ought to think that we are one of the leaves of a tree,
and the tree is all humanity.

Pablo Casals

THERE IS NO clear dividing line between the animal and the human mind. Instead of a "first human," there was a gradual progression from one way of experiencing the world to another. The many similarities between our behavior and those of lower primates clearly demonstrate how our more primitive natures were conserved alongside our later-evolving abilities. Many of the structures and functions of our mammalian ancestors are conserved within our modern brains.

We know that the expansion of the cortex in primates corresponds with ever growing social groups. There is not only safety in numbers but also the ability for task specialization, such as hunting, gathering, and caretaking. So while many animals need to be born immediately prepared to take on the challenges of survival, human infants have the luxury of years of total dependency during which our brains can slowly be shaped by very specific environments. Relationships are a fundamental and necessary condition for the existence of the contemporary human brain.

To more deeply appreciate how our brains learn, we have to utilize a variety of disciplines, including evolutionary biology, social psychology, cultural anthropology, and genetics. Through these and other sciences, we can learn about patterns of instinctual and unconscious behaviors as well as witness them in action across a variety of living cultures. Each discipline provides us with a glimpse of the emerging patterns of humanity through the thousand generations that connect the beginning of our written history to our ancient animal ancestry.

Successful social behavior required increasingly complex brains, and complex brains required more help from other brains to develop, organize, and stay on track. Eventually, this double helix of complexity and sociality wove families and tribes into **superorganisms**—a word used to describe a group made up of many individuals who serve collective survival. The more social our brains became, the more important relationships became as sociostatic regulators of our minds, bodies, and emotions. For those of you familiar with systems therapy, this is nothing new.

Definition: Superorganism

A superorganism is an organism consisting of many organisms that cooperate for mutual survival. Social animals and insects are the commonly cited examples. Within a superorganism, the environment and the group both come to serve as evolutionary selection variables. That is, the individual is shaped by his or her contribution to the group while the groups are shaped to match the natural environment.

Two consequences of human evolution seem particularly relevant to both the birth and success of psychotherapy. The first is that we evolved into social animals who are highly attuned to one another's inner experiences. This sympathetic attunement allows us to influence each other's thoughts, feelings, and behaviors. The second is that our attachment circuitry remains plastic throughout life. If you have any doubts about this, just ask grandparents how they feel about their grandchildren. Through the new science of epigenetics, we now know that we participate in the way each other's brains are built, how they develop, and how they function.

As social animals we possess strong instincts to connect, and our brains have been wired to love and contribute to our tribe. In other words, we want to love and be loved, have a successful career, and be well thought of by others. So if we are having relationships, making babies, being creative, and living up to our potential, we will probably not seek therapy. These people are linked to the group mind and can use their social connections to process and heal life's bruises naturally, much as a cut naturally forms a scab and heals over time. The need for psychotherapy arises when the social connections are absent, distorted, or damaged due to trauma, depression, or other challenges.

Nurturance and Survival

> *Being deeply loved gives you strength, while loving someone deeply*
> *gives you courage.*
> Lao Tzu

Our first months of life are dedicated to getting to know our mother: her smell, taste, feel, and the look of her face. We gradually experience her ability to attune to us and soothe our distress as her presence becomes synonymous with safety. As we grow, our mothers and fathers shape our brains from the inside out in a dance of interacting instincts. For a human baby, survival doesn't depend on how fast it can run, whether it can climb a tree, or if it can tell the difference between edible and poisonous mushrooms. Rather, we survive based on our abilities to detect the needs and intentions of those around us. For humans, other people are our primary environment. If we are successful in relationships, we will have food, shelter, protection, and children of our own. We get what we need through our interdependence with others, which is why abandonment is equated with death in the mind of a child.

In contemporary society, adults are required to multitask, balance the demands of work and family, manage a vast amount of information, and cope with stress. We need to maintain perspective, pick our battles carefully, and remain mindful of ourselves in the midst of countless competing demands. What prepares us best for these abilities? In some ways, it is the same thing that prepared our ancestors to survive in their world: early nurturance, which plays a vital role in the development and integration of the diverse systems within our brains. Optimal sculpting of the prefrontal cortex through healthy early relationships allows us to think well of ourselves, trust others, regulate our emotions, maintain positive expectations, and utilize our intellectual and emotional intelligence in moment-to-moment problem solving. We can now add a corollary to Darwin's theory of natural selection: those who are nurtured best, survive best in a complex social world.

When parents neglect, abandon, or are consistently mis-attuned to their children, the parent is communicating to the child that he is less fit. This is not intentional, but a by-product of how very young brains process information. Consequently, the child's brain may become shaped in ways that do not support his long-term survival. Nonloving behavior signals to children that the world is a dangerous place and tells them "do not explore, do not discover, and most of all, do not take chances." When children are traumatized, abused, or neglected, they grow up to have thoughts, states of mind, emotions, and immunological functioning that are incongruent with health and long-term survival. In other words, what doesn't kill us makes us weaker.

Maternal and paternal instincts, in fact all caretaking behaviors, are acts of nurturance that trump one's personal survival. Achieving such an altruistic state depends upon the successful inhibition of selfish, competitive, and aggressive impulses. Too often, however, that inhibition is incomplete. The fact that we spend so much time in psychotherapy dealing with the impact of our relationships with our parents reflects that our evolution as caretakers is still a work in progress.

Clients love to complain about their partners, but it is also important to keep in mind that everyone is married to the wrong person. I don't mean that everyone makes a bad choice when choosing a mate, but that everyone expects from their partner what their partner is unable to provide—being the parent they've always wanted. Because of this, we always end up resenting who we are with because we compare them to another who might have been able to do it right. This fantasy is wrapped around the wish to be heard, seen, felt, and understood as you have always needed to be. We can help our mates do this better for us, but they will never live up to the fantasy.

Human Apoptosis: Programmed Self-Destruction

> *When God desires to destroy a thing, he entrusts its destruction*
> *to the thing itself.*
> Victor Hugo

The internal logic of our social brains rests on a principle that goes back to the beginning of the universe. When different molecules touch, they bond together in a manner that increases the diversity, complexity, and adaptive capacity of matter. For example, water exists because two hydrogen and one oxygen molecule combine to form one water molecule (H_2O). This logic continued after the emergence of organic compounds, when single-celled organisms combined to created multicellular organisms of increasing diversity and complexity. As colonies of complex cells became the main unit of survival, individual cells were programmed to either connect and contribute, or die.

We see this in the development of the brain, where many of the cells we are born with die during development. We are born with many more cells than we need, like a large block of marble brought to a sculptor's studio. The sculptor's job is to find the statue within the block of marble by removing those pieces that don't contribute to the final product. In a similar way, experience shapes the functional networks of the brain through strengthening connections between cells that became wired together in the execution of functional tasks. Those cells that do not contribute are not stimulated and eventually die off in a process called apoptosis. This is not a pathological process but a normal part of brain development. In fact, individuals with autism often show a failure of apoptosis and have a higher density of neurons. Thus, the sacrifice of some neurons is important for the survival of the many.

Neuroscience Corner: Apoptosis

As the brain is shaped by experience, neurons that do not contribute to functional networks die and are cleaned away by glial cells. This process, called apoptosis, is a normal and necessary aspect of brain growth. A failure of normal apoptosis will contribute to dysfunctions of mental processing.

Just as brains are composed of cells, tribes are made up of individual people. In subsistence tribes, individuals who cannot contribute to the tribe's survival—the infirm, the elderly, and those born with deformities—were most often killed or allowed to die. In some cultures, it is a woman's job to kill her newborn if it suffers from any obvious birth defects. Without extra resources to care for those who cannot carry their own weight, challenged individuals put the rest of the tribe at risk.

There is an interesting parallel to apoptosis in human experience, which has been referred to as failure to thrive or **anaclitic depression**. The Austrian psychiatrist René Spitz noticed that infants orphaned by the Nazi blitz showed an initial phase of protest and bursts of activity, followed by a loss of energy and the appearance of deflation, often followed by death. Like infants, neurons strive to connect with other neurons and activate bursts of energy as they attempt to connect. If they are shunned by other neurons, they eventually run out of steam and die. My suggestion is that when humans are cut off from their primary sources of attachment, we are programed to wither and die the same way neurons do.

The fact that suicidal ideation and suicide attempts are often triggered by breakups, separation, and death has strengthened my conviction that apoptosis is an appropriate model for human experience. Suicide is also motivated by being socially shamed, such as in situations of bankruptcy, criminal convictions, and other losses of face. Suicidal patients often report childhoods they experienced as being lonely, disconnected, and unloving. Finally, and perhaps most convincing, is that the clients who struggle with depression often respond very well to having their suicidal urges interpreted as expressions of loneliness and a need for reattunement.

Definition: Anaclitic Depression

Anaclitic depression, also called hospitalism, is a wasting disease in infancy caused by a lack of social contact with caretakers. First noticed in children in hospitals and orphanages, it led to changes to increase interaction and contact for institutionalized infants and children. I interpret this as a direct parallel to the process of apoptosis in neurons.

After establishing a secure connection, the most important thing to create with clients is a language for their internal experiences. It is best if this language contains objective symptoms that allow them to put some distance between their thoughts and emotions. When a symptom is experienced as separate from the self, it can eventually become something capable of being discarded or forcibly expelled. Thus, a potential benefit of thinking of the brain as a social organ is learning to interpret self-destructive urges as indications of disconnection. The inner feeling associated with shame is essentially an internalized message that we are unwanted, unnecessary, and even detrimental to the tribe.

Embedded within what Freud called the superego (the internalization of parents' attitude toward the self) is a message of whether parents felt you should live or die—were you wanted or unwanted, were you a benefit or hindrance to the life of the family or tribe? Should you live or be killed? Although our clients do not have any explicit memory of their early relationships with their parents, these experiences are implicitly recorded in how the patients think about and treat themselves. The negativity in our self-image and the way we treat ourselves sometimes exposes our parents' negative or indifferent attitudes toward us decades earlier. Many with urges to harm or kill themselves were programmed within primitive memory systems before they were old enough to remember learning anything. Our own value and lovability are among the lessons that we don't remember learning, but never forget.

Jury Dismissed

> *Throughout evolution, ostracism was death indeed.*
> Helen Fisher

I'd been seeing David for about three months when he came in with a faraway look, a stark contrast to his usually cheerful presentation. He seemed to be deeper within himself today; I let him sit quietly for a while before I asked what was on his mind. David looked right at me with an expression I had never seen on him before, both happy and frightened at the same time. Finally he spoke.

"I've had a revelation this week. I realized that I've lived my life with a courtroom inside my head. Everywhere I go, whatever I do, there is a parallel drama going on inside of me—I am the defendant on trial, and I know that even though I am innocent, I will be found guilty. Because the verdict is predetermined, the trial feels pro forma. I know instinctually that the trial will never end, but at the same time, anticipating the guilty verdict is torture. I don't remember not being on trial; it seems like it started when I was very young, and I just came to take it for granted. I unwittingly assumed that everyone lives their lives on trial. Do they? Do you?"

David continued, "You know when you are awakened from a dream and for awhile, you are both awake and in the dream? That's what its like—two stories interwoven into one. In fact, it's happening right now. I'm sitting across from you, and intellectually I know that you like me and accept me for who I am. In all the time I've known you, you've never criticized or attacked me, never used me or taken advantage of me. You've always done your best for me. That's one story line.

"But despite that, I sit here and expect you to criticize and abandon me. When you begin to speak, and then hesitate, in that split second my mind makes up all of these ideas about what you are going to say, like, 'You are just too boring for me to work with, so I need to refer you to another therapist,' or 'There are other people who deserve my time more than you do.' So while I trust you, the voice in my head is sure you will abandon me."

This is a heartbreakingly beautiful description of early shame programming in systems of implicit memory. It is also a clear example of our brain's ability to provide the mind with two simultaneous realities. Because one role of implicit memory is to use past experience to anticipate and control current situations, past shaming experiences prime conscious awareness to anticipate rejection. This courtroom scenario is reminiscent of Dostoyevsky's *Crime and Punishment*, where the main character is haunted by the anticipation of condemnation.

After many years of intense work focused on rooting out and fighting against shame, David gradually became aware that his inner world had changed. His courtroom had been remodeled through a combination of reality testing, experimenting with visibility, and creative visual imagery. "Over time I've dismissed the judge and jury and removed the bench and the jury box. For the most part, I don't experience my life through the eyes of others, and I'm aware of my feelings, needs, and predilections.

"The jury box has been replaced with a comfortable sitting area that I use as a kind of meditation space to go to throughout the day. It has a mirror and some candles around it that give off a soft glow. I look into this mirror and check in with myself, reflecting on my emotions and what I feel in my body. I remember to breathe and check to see if I'm tense or upset about something. I know this sounds self-centered but it is actually the self-nurturing I need in order to be with people. What I used to do looked more social because I was obsessively focused on other people, but it wasn't about them. It was all about my fear of rejection. Now I can actually pay attention to others because I can stop being preoccupied with myself."

If children don't get help to understand how to articulate their inner experiences, be aware of their needs, and feel like they have a right to be taken care of, all of life can become an act performed to a hostile audience. Turning that around to live from the inside out is the work of managing and potentially healing shame. Children who don't experience proper attunement project their self-identities behind the eyes of other people. They live in exile from themselves and see themselves as they think others see them—almost always as bad. They strive for perfection to avoid rejection.

While I've never felt that I have completely banished core shame for any of my clients, the change in this narrative made me feel that we had come close. "From time to time when I look in the mirror, instead of seeing myself, I see a judge or a juror. Those memories are still inside of me and seem to reappear when I feel stressed or rejected by someone. Fortunately, they appear less and less frequently, and I am more quickly able to realize what is happening and reconnect with my own image."

Core shame is more like diabetes than a cold, something to manage rather than something we get over. The programming may just be too deeply embedded in our brains to completely remove. Like getting over fears and phobias, we can only build new neural networks to inhibit the expression of the symptoms.

Self-Harm, Suicidal Gestures, and the Rage of Abandonment

A suicide kills two people, Maggie, that's what it's for!
Arthur Miller

Clients who engage in repeated self-harm almost always describe childhoods that include abuse, neglect, or cruel teasing at the hands of parents and/or caretakers. This suggests that some cases of self-harm may be triggered by intrusive memories of early attachment relationships activated by criticism, rejection, and loss. Many clients will automatically and unconsciously translate these feelings into self-injurious or suicidal acts, which can be reinforced by the subsequent attention of professionals, family, and friends.

Both the self-harm and the resulting attention can become a means of affect regulation that parallels the distress calls of primates whose oxytocin levels drop in the absence of the mother. The reappearance of the mother (or the rescuers of the self-destructive client) raises oxytocin levels, calming the infant. In case of injury, endorphins provide analgesia for pain to allow us to continue to fight or flee. Endorphin and oxytocin levels rise and fall and rise again in both infant and mother as they draw near one another, separate, and reunite. These neuroendocrine reactions and their role in the modulation of proximity may be central to the experiences and behaviors of clients identified with borderline symptoms. These patients report less maternal protectiveness in childhood, which correlates with more stress and higher cortisol levels. It has also been found that suicide attempts in borderline personality disorder are more likely to have interpersonal triggers than in depressed patients.

In most individuals, release of endogenous endorphins in response to fear and stress may help modulate emotional states and enhance coping and problem solving. The analgesic effects of these morphine-like substances may also account for the reports of reduced anxiety and a sense of calm after cutting or burning. Research has demonstrated that self-harm decreases or terminates completely when patients are given a drug to block the effects of endogenous opioids. In individuals with borderline personality disorder, this system may not become activated under normal conditions, and self-harm might be a way to move past a higher threshold for endorphin release.

It is difficult to treat clients who are self-injurious or suicidal because of our dual responsibilities to encourage their growth into the future and to keep them alive in the moment. Usually, the focus on growth is eclipsed by the panic created in us by their dangerous actions. As much as you care for your client, it is difficult not to catastrophize being blamed, being sued, losing your license, or being crushed by a lifetime of guilt. In a state of panic, it is difficult to stay cortical, think straight, problem solve, and come up with good ideas.

The goal of therapy with clients who are suicidal or self-harming is to get them to replace self-destructive acts with more adaptive behaviors. Because I believe that self-harm is an expression of fear of abandonment and loss, my goal is to replace self-destructive acts with naming and sharing the feelings that trigger them.

Turning Self-Harm Into Self-Expression

When in trouble, disclose on the double.

Gerald Goodman

As I was leaving the office one Friday evening, I noticed that the light on my phone was blinking. Usually, I would have kept going and picked up the message later, but for some reason, I decided to answer the call. When I picked up the phone, I heard lots of noise on the other end and a man's voice telling me that he was going to kill himself. As I concentrated on his voice, I recognized him as John, a client that I had been working with for the past few months who suffered with chronic depression, social isolation, and erratic interpersonal behaviors. What I could make out was that John was in his car and that he had decided to end his life. He just wanted to say goodbye and thank me for all of my help.

My immediate reaction was panic—OMG! What am I going to do?—as the child in my head ran around in circles. The next set of thoughts focused on calming myself down and obtaining more information.

I was able to learn that John was in his garage with his engine running, and I deduced through all of the noise that he was trying to kill himself with the fumes. I probably didn't have much time to act, and even if I had another phone to call the police in his town, they would never get there in time to save him—it was up to me. Nothing in my training had prepared me for this scenario, so I had to navigate on instinct. I assumed that if John was calling me, he was ambivalent about dying. I also assumed that if he was calling me to thank me for trying to help him, then the real message was "Fuck you for not doing a better job." Based on these two ideas, here is what I did.

I made believe that it was much more difficult to hear him than it actually was and kept asking him to repeat certain words. I finally asked John if he could turn off the car so I could make out what he was saying, which he did. This is when the real conversation began.

Rather than focus on the suicidal behavior, I asked him what feeling he had been having that day. Alternating between talking and coughing, John told me that was feeling lonely and hopeless and that he didn't feel like I was taking his pain seriously. It was true that he presented much better externally than he felt inside, and I probably responded too much to his presentation instead of his suffering. I apologized for not having heard him and expressed that I wanted to try to be a better therapist. I eventually suggested that he open the garage door because his coughing was making it difficult to understand everything he was saying.

So, at multiple levels, I kept the conversation focused on the quality of our attachment and my failures of attunement to John instead of focusing on the suicidal gesture. This is based on my idea that the self-destructive act is itself triggered by abandonment and that while my immediate goal is to keep my clients alive, the long-term goal is to get them to connect and heal. Unfortunately, the focus of our field is all about the act instead of its meaning. My experience is that clients continue to be self-destructive until they come to feel seen, heard, and felt.

The fact that it was beyond my control to intervene in any physical way made this strategy my only leverage. This interaction proved to be one of the many nodal points of therapy that took us step-by-step from an avoidant to a secure attachment relationship that then served as a platform for healing. The truth is that if someone really wants to kill himself, he will be able to do it. Part of the risk of being a therapist is that we will end up working with a suicidal client who will succeed no matter how well we do our job. It is something we have to accept and learn to live with. I doubt that any therapist who has had a client commit suicide is ever the same. More important, however, is the fact that we will help most of our clients through the darkness of depression to a life that will be worth living.

CHAPTER 7

Attachment and
Intimate Relationships

The greatest happiness of life is the conviction that we are loved.
Victor Hugo

THE POWER OF secure attachment is at the core of all nurturing, supportive, and healing relationships. It is therefore easy to understand why aspects of friendship, mentoring, and parenting all appear during successful psychotherapy. While secure attachments can take many forms, they all share a minimum of criticism, competition, and conflict. Feeling accepted by others is a profound experience, resulting in states of brain and mind that enhance neuroplasticity and positive change. This is why the Rogerian cornerstones of caring, empathy, and positive regard have remained central to our field through hundreds of therapeutic fads and new techniques.

One of the primary reasons I appreciate a neuroscientific approach to therapy is that in the eyes of science, both therapist and client are bipedal primates with flawed brains. The humility and vulnerability this perspective brings to therapy supports the establishment of a secure attachment. Engaging in a shared struggle to make up for some of evolution's less brilliant choices levels the playing field in a nice way. As a therapist, it reminds me that I struggle with many of the same challenges and conflicts for which my clients come to me for help. We are all in this together. Safety is at the heart of positive change. If therapists can put aside their need for status, their intellectual agenda, and their personal struggles for a while, they can create an interpersonal matrix of change. If clients have the strength and the courage to be accepted and explore their inner worlds, they can join in this connection in ways that may lead to insight and healing. If both can admit that they are just two people trying to make it through the day and that the roles of client and therapist don't imply status or power, there is hope.

What Is Attachment?

For small creatures such as we, the vastness is bearable only through love.
Carl Sagan

Attachment is an evolutionary strategy to keep parents and children close. Attachment emerged during natural selection because proximity enhanced the survival of children and, hence, the survival of the group. The same biological levers were utilized with tribes as larger and more coherent groups increased the odds of survival. At the core of attachment circuitry is the amygdala, our organ of appraisal and the executive center of fear processing.

When parents and children are close, they both feel safer and calmer and experience a general sense of well-being. When separated, parents and children become distressed as their amygdala signal danger. This triggers parents to search and call out and children to emit distress calls to make their location known. When reunited, their chemistry shifts as they transition from a sense of fear to safety.

Like all biological organisms, we are constantly shifting from states of homeostatic balance to imbalance and back again. We become hungry and eventually eat; we become frightened and eventually find safety; we become cranky and tired and eventually fall asleep. These are all examples of a pattern of going from regulation, to dysregulation, to reregulation, which our brains summarize and use for future reference as they make connections and construct conscious experience.

During infancy and childhood, we have a vast number of experiences of going from being safe and calm to feeling distressed and endangered. We are sleeping soundly, only to wake up hungry, wet, or needing to be burped; we are joyfully running through the kitchen, only to fall and bump our heads; we wander into a room and become terrified by the unexpected darkness. In each of these situations we cry out in confusion, pain, or fear. We have gone from a state of calm or positive excitement to one of upset and fear.

If we are dysregulated as infants, we reflexively cry out to summon our parents. If the caretaker arrives and we move to a state of regulation, our primitive brain circuitry pairs the presence of the other with positive emotion. So in reality, we may have been crying out because our wet diaper was burning our skin. After a successful change, we now feel comfortable, smell better, and have experienced some positive sights, sounds, and touches from our mom or dad. This is a piece of building secure attachment—the association of the arrival of another with a shift to a positive state of body, emotion, and mind. As the theory goes, if we have enough of these positive associations to the presence of others, we have a good chance of having a secure attachment.

The opposite occurs when we are dysregulated and the

arrival of the other either doesn't lead to reregulation or, even worse, increases our dysregulation. So in the above example, if we are crying out and no one arrives, or if they add to our distress by screaming at us for annoying them, we will not associate the arrival of the other with reregulation. We may even come to associate the other with an increase in distress. A preponderance of these experiences may lead to an insecure attachment style. People with insecure attachment styles lack the ability to be soothed by others in a consistent and predictable way. Overall, the difference between a secure and insecure attachment style is this—secure attachments help to regulate arousal and anxiety while insecure attachments do not.

Attachment theory is based on the assumption that these experiences are stored in systems of implicit memory. Are others attentive to our distress, able to discern what has happened and to bring us back to a state of calm and safety? Or are they unavailable, unattuned to our needs, or unable to make us feel better? Our early experiences with caretakers shape our predictions of the ability of others to soothe our distress and make us feel safe. These implicit memory patterns, or attachment schema, so named by John Bowlby, are activated in future intimate relationships and shape the way we experience and relate to others.

Attachment Schema

> *We can only learn to love by loving.*
> Alice Murdock

An attachment schema is essentially a pattern of expectation established within us about the ability of other people to help us feel safe. Four categories of attachment schema have emerged from research: (1) secure, (2) avoidant, (3) anxious-ambivalent, and (4) insecure-disorganized. The descriptions that follow are general tendencies observed in children and their mothers in these four categories.

1. Securely attached children have parents who are good at being available and are attuned to their children's' needs. They have the ability to fluidly switch their attention from what they are doing to their child and to disconnect when they are no longer needed. When distressed, their children seek proximity, are quickly soothed, and return to exploration and play. These children seem to expect their caretakers to be attentive, helpful, and encouraging of their continued autonomy. It is believed that they have learned that when they are distressed, interacting with their mothers will help them to regain a sense of security.
2. Avoidantly attached children tend to have caretakers who are inattentive and dismissive of them and their needs. When these children are under stress, they either ignore their parents or just glance at them without engagement. Despite their anxiety, these children lack the expectation that their parents are a source of soothing and seem to have learned that it is easier to be self-reliant and regulate their own emotions.
3. Anxious-ambivalent children have enmeshed or inconsistently available caregivers. They seek proximity when distressed, but they are not easily soothed and are slow to return to play. In many cases, their distress seems to be worsened by their mothers' anxiety and uncertainty. These children tend

to cling more and engage in less exploration, as if they have learned from their mothers' anxiety that the world is a dangerous place and better to be avoided.

4. Children with disorganized attachment, when under stress, appear to have a conflictual relationship with their mothers. They want to approach to be soothed while at the same time appear to be afraid to approach. It is as if they are experiencing an internal approach-avoidance conflict that is reflected in chaotic and even self-injurious behaviors; they spin, fall down, hit themselves, and don't know what to do to calm themselves. They appear to dissociate and are overcome by trancelike expressions, freeze in place, or maintain uncomfortable bodily postures. It has been found that disorganized attachment in children correlates with unresolved grief and/or trauma in their mothers, which makes them both frightened and frightening to their children.

Humans love categories, especially ones that foster a sense of understanding and certainty. Attachment researchers have spent a half century exploring, articulating, and confirming the validity of these categories. From this perspective, it is easy to think of them as distinct and well-defined ways of connecting (or not) in close relationships. But as a psychotherapist, my primary concern has been to understand how I can assist individuals with insecure and disorganized patterns of attachment to gain security and change categories. From this perspective, therapists are far more interested in the fluctuations and instability of attachment schema. So the big question is, do the neural systems of implicit memory that encode attachment schema remain plastic?

Attachment Plasticity

> *There is no remedy for love but to love more.*
> Henry David Thoreau

Research with other social mammals has demonstrated patterns of mother-child interaction similar to what we see in humans. This research strongly suggests that both the intrauterine environment and maternal behavior after birth serve as mechanisms that shape brain development in the direction of adaptation to specific environmental conditions. For example, mothers who live in the presence of more danger build their children's brains in ways that lead them to be less exploratory and more vigilant. In other words, both their biochemistry and their behavior become a template upon which their babies' brains are sculpted. In this manner, the fetus and infant get a heads-up that they had better be ready for danger.

It thus appears that the transmission of stress to the fetus, infant, and juvenile shapes adaptational patterns matched to the type of environment they will be facing. There is also evidence that when the environment becomes less stressful, patterns of behavior shape a greater sense of security. In humans, more insecure children are born to mothers in areas with fewer resources and more violence. It appears that nature is preparing these children for the world they will have to survive in.

If attachment schema are adaptational strategies that can change with environmental changes, then one of our main objectives in therapy is to assist those who are unable to feel safe with others to learn to do so. After all, the ability to love is not only one of life's main objectives, it also allows us to benefit from the naturally healthful impacts of positive relationships.

Despite the evidence of an attachment schema by our first birthday, research strongly suggests that it is not set in neural stone. These naturally occurring changes and the fact that we attach and reattach with many people throughout our lives suggests that the underlying neural systems maintain their plasticity. In support of the neuroplasticity of attachment networks, adults can create secure attachment for their children despite negative experiences in their own childhoods.

The flexibility of schema reflects the underlying reality that attachment schema are survival strategies that can be modified in the face of new experience. It appears that if someone who is insecurely attached is lucky enough to stick with a securely attached person for about five years, it increases her own attachment security. I suspect that you would find a similar change in the other direction for secure individuals who end up with someone who treats them badly. The stress of negative events and relationships operate to maintain insecure attachment by continuing to send danger signals to the amygdala and the networks it controls. Secure attachment, while not impervious, appears more resistant to change than insecure attachment.

Thus, the powerful shaping of childhood can be modified through personal relationships, psychotherapy, and/or experiences that increase self-awareness. The ability to consciously process stressful and traumatic life events appears to correlate with more secure attachment, flexible affect regulation, and an increased availability of narrative memory. A healing relationship with a secure partner or with a good-enough therapist, in which past fears can be processed and resolved, can help us to achieve secure attachment schema. The major implication for psychotherapy from all of these findings is that insecure attachment is subject to change as a result of positive connectivity.

As a psychotherapist interested in positive change, I want attachment schema to be a changeable form of implicit memory so relationships with clients can alter them in a salubrious manner. In this way, psychotherapy can become a guided attachment relationship for the purposes of assisted emotional regulation and the eventual adjustment of insecure schema. Most importantly, intergeneration patterns of maltreatment and insecure attachment can be disrupted with the proper professional interventions or personal experiences.

Attachment in Psychotherapy

The first duty of love is to listen.
Paul Tillich

Clients who come to therapy with the ability to develop secure attachment bonds are able to use us relatively quickly to regulate their anxiety. That is, they join in the creation of a dyadic organism (therapist and client) and are able to use the therapist's brain to regulate their own. This will happen as a natural outgrowth of time spent together and the accumulation of positive interactions.

Clients who are insecurely attached may be sitting in the same seat with the same issues and even saying the same words, but they are watching the therapist from the other side of a protective screen. They established these defenses long ago to protect themselves from the pain and disappointment of a lack of availability, care, and emotional attunement from others. These are the clients who are often said to have personality disorders.

So, the big question: how do you help someone who is insecurely attached to develop a secure attachment with you? And how do you overwrite the memories of their first parenting experiences with a new set of experiences based on your abilities to be consistent, present, and attuned? Wouldn't it be great if there were a simple and straightforward manual for that?

Just like parenting the first time, reparenting is long and difficult, with many bumps along the way. It takes a lot of patience and emotional regulation on the part of the therapist. It's the client's job (unconsciously of course) to get you to respond to them the way their parents did. If they expect rejection, they will make themselves worthy of rejection. If they expect to have their boundaries violated by being seduced, they will make themselves available for violation, act seductively, and become angry whether you do or don't live up to their expectations. In a sense, the client's job is to take you hostage into their past and your job is to elude capture, while naming what is happening and remaining supportive in the process. Thinking in terms of these three steps may be helpful:

Step 1: You have to be the parent they didn't have—someone who is present, stays attuned to them, and respects their perspective. The goal of this is to get to the point in the relationship when clients realize that they continue to use their defenses even though they are no longer necessary —Carl Rogers was great at this.

Step 2: When a true connection is established, sadness and grief often emerge. These emotions are reactions to having not gotten what they needed during childhood and to the realization that their defensive reactions have kept them from getting these things in adulthood. This grief period should be attuned to and encouraged but after awhile, you should encourage clients to begin with new experiments in living. Remind them from time to time that grief is a stage, not a lifestyle. This is not an emotional state that you want them to become trapped in.

Step 3: The real neural reshaping process occurs during experiments in living after new ways of connecting and interacting with others are discussed. Each client with an insecure attachment history will have a long list of past social behaviors that had negative outcomes. The first stage is to stop doing the things that don't work. As clients experiment with new behaviors, therapy becomes the crucible for planning and post hoc analysis of new ways of interacting. The biggest challenges that you can help clients with are their faulty and shame-based thoughts, emotions, and behaviors. The second stage is to help clients deal with the anxiety of taking on the experiments and working with techniques for stress reduction, such as meditation, yoga, or whatever means they can use to downregulate amygdala activation.

It's helpful to think of insecure attachment as a form of posttraumatic memory, not resistance. This makes it easier to avoid blaming clients for their behavior and helps the therapist to avoid feeling rejected. Although we don't like to admit it, therapists get hurt by "noncooperative" clients. Thus, in their personal therapy, therapists should explore their own need to be loved, appreciated, and listened to.

Building Inhibitory Circuits From the Cortex to the Amygdala

Love cures people—both the ones who give it and the ones who receive it.

Karl Menninger

So what is the mechanism of action that changes insecure to secure attachment? How do repeated cycles of attunement, misattunement, and reattunement result in our ability to regulate stress and stay connected in the face of anxiety and fear? Kohut used the term transmuting internalizations to describe this process—very poetic, but what does it mean?

The amygdala is at the core of fear circuitry. Based on our current findings in neuroscience, it is believed that our amygdala have evolved to store negative associations on a permanent basis. Insecure attachment schema have, at their core, an association within the amygdala of fear, negative experiences, and emotional dysregulation paired with intimate relationships. So as much as someone may desire intimacy, the amygdala activates a danger signal, triggering autonomic arousal and a fight-flight response to closeness. This pairing needs to be inhibited if a secure attachment relationship is to be established.

When we overcome fears and phobias, heal from posttraumatic stress, or move from insecure to secure attachment schema, we are building new neural systems or reinforcing those already in place. These systems will most likely include descending inhibitory circuits from the prefrontal cortex down to the amygdala. Although we think of the cortex as primarily excitatory and a storehouse of our memories and knowledge, its role as an inhibitor is just as important. Here is a good example of its inhibitory role.

Neuroscience Corner: Descending Inhibition

The ability of the cortex to inhibit limbic midbrain and brain stem structures, allowing us to inhibit early reflexes and learned fear responses stored in these regions.

My son was handed to me by a nurse about 30 seconds after he was born. I stared at him as he struggled to open his eyes to make sense of the world. He was worn out from passing through an all-too-small birth canal, and I was nearly delirious from sleep deprivation and the terrors of fatherhood. The nurse pointed to the other side of the birthing room to a small Plexiglas box, indicating where I was to put him. Luckily, I made it across the room without falling and placed all six pounds of him on a thin blanket inside the plastic box.

A couple of feet above his head were heat lamps that reminded me of the ones that keep the French fries warm at McDonald's. Of course, the lights were bright and they must have been especially bright for eyes that were a minute old. So I held my left hand above his face to protect his eyes from the glare. Within seconds, he reached up with his tiny right hand and grabbed my pinky and then with his left and grabbed my thumb, and pulled my hand down onto his face. Now I understand that this is a primitive brain stem reflex and has nothing to do with children recognizing and loving their parents. But of course, this was my child, not some anonymous child in a textbook, and I felt sure that he recognized me and was telling me that he loved me. So much for scientific objectivity. This primitive grasping reflex, also known as the Palmar grasp, is controlled by the brain stem. It is believed to be an evolutionary holdover from when baby primates had to hold onto the fur of their mothers as they moved about and took care of business. I've seen it in action in newborns and infants. You can place your fingers against their palms, triggering them to clamp on. Their grasp is so strong that they can actually be lifted up in this way well into their second and third month of life. I had always assumed that this ability was lost when they became too heavy to hold themselves; turns out I was wrong.

What happens in those first few months is that the cortex sends descending fibers down to actively inhibit this brain stem reflex. The reason the cortex does this so early in development is to free the hands up from this primitive grasping reflex so that the motor areas in the cortex can take over the hands and turn them from a primitive pair of pliers into an orchestra of ten dexterous fingers. Here's another interesting piece of the puzzle involving descending cortical inhibition.

When my son grows to be an old man and if he shows some signs of memory loss or confusion, his children may take him to a neurologist for an exam. When the neurologist examines him, she will ask him to hold his arms outstretched with his palms down. She will then slide her fingers along the bottom of his arms, starting at the elbow and moving toward his hands. When she gets to his hands, she will cup her fingers a bit to stimulate his palms to see if her touch causes a grasp reflex. If it does, it will be an indication that my son, now in his old age, may be beginning to lose neurons in his frontal and temporal lobes.

But why would the grasp reflex come back? Because it was being actively inhibited for decades to free up the hands to be used for writing and playing the piano. As the cortical neurons dedicated to inhibiting it after birth begin to die because of dementia, the brain stem once again asserts the power of the Palmar grasp. In neurology, this is called a cortical release sign—the return of these reflexes reflects a compromised cortex. The truth is, the Palmar reflex was there the entire time but actively inhibited by descending cortical circuits.

Neuroscience Corner: Cortical Release Sign

The return of a primitive reflex later in life that reflects damage to a region of the cortex that has been dedicated to inhibiting it. Cortical release signs are often an indication of some form of brain injury or disease.

I tell you this story not because you plan on being a neurologist, but because it is important in understanding the mechanism of action of helping clients move from an insecure to a secure attachment. Just like the inhibition of the Palmar reflex, the cortex also sends descending fibers to the amygdala to influence its activation in response to the world. When we are able to assist a client to get over a fear of intimacy, we have actually built new neural connections that are inhibiting the amygdala's ability to activate our fight-flight response in relationships.

So when we are going through the repetitive cycles of regulation, dysregulation, and reregulation with our clients, we are remodeling the attachment circuitry that they came to therapy with. Every time clients have a negative expectation of us—such as criticizing, shaming, or abandoning them—a new and more positive memory is being added into the mix. The skills we give them to downregulate their anxiety allow them to remain self-reflective and stimulate more cortical activation, leading to the building and remodeling of new descending fibers. The more cortical activation they can maintain in the face of stress, the more emotional regulation they will develop.

Like helicopter parents, all our amygdala want to do is protect us from any potential harm. They scare the hell out of us to keep us out of harm's way. Unfortunately, an overprotective amygdala can make life not worth living. By seemingly endless cycles of regulation, dysregulation, and reregulation, therapists, like parents, can build new cortical circuitry to convince the amygdala that we have nothing to fear. What is transmuted in the process of therapy is the strength, coherence, and connectivity of neural circuits that allow us to inhibit fears programmed decades before and learn new, more adaptive ways of being.

CHAPTER 8

Core Shame

The worst loneliness is to not be comfortable with yourself.

Mark Twain

ALL OF US are born exploding with primitive, selfish, and uncivilized instincts—a part of our psyche Freud called the id. We expect to be the center of attention and have our parents' complete and undivided attention. Because caretakers work hard to provide for our every physical and emotional need during the first year of life, this fantasy is, at first, largely fulfilled. However, as children begin to explore their environments, they are exposed to a dangerous world. We are taught shame to keep us safe, but it is a visceral reminder of how dependent we are. As a result, we react to an emotional threat as though our physical survival depends on it.

This freeze response is coded within the autonomic nervous system as a rapid transition from sympathetic arousal to parasympathetic inhibition. When the freeze response is triggered, children are snapped from a mode of curiosity and exploration to one of fear, rigidity, and withdrawal. As a result, the child stops, looks downward, hangs his head, and rounds his shoulders. The consequences of this primitive form of social control become central in both intimate relationships and how we behave in groups. If you were going to design a mechanism of social control that would keep alphas in line behind betas, you couldn't do better than core shame. Those with core shame try to be perfect soldiers and only feel confident when they are following someone else's orders.

Bad Dog!

The disappearance of a sense of responsibility is the most far-reaching consequence of submission to authority.
Stanley Milgram

If you scold your dog for soiling the rug or chewing up the sofa, he will hunch over and roll over on his back, or pull his tail between his legs and slink away. Similar postures occur in reaction to exclusion, judgment, and submission in virtually all social animals. It essentially says "You're the boss."

Most children aren't overly damaged by this social conditioning; after all, we have to absorb plenty of corrections during life. Although we all want to be kings and queens of the world, our parents want respectful, hard-working, and well-behaved children. Problems in psychological and intellectual development can occur, however, when a child is met with prolonged scolding, criticism, and rejection. This can occur due to harsh parenting, oversensitive children, and a variety of other factors that can thwart the development of healthy self-esteem. The overuse of shame as a disciplinary tool also predisposes children to longterm difficulties with emotional regulation. Chronically shaming parents have children who spend much of their time anxious, afraid, and at risk for depression and anxiety.

An important aspect of avoiding instilling core shame is to

rescue children from withdrawn and dysregulated states by reattuning with them as soon as possible after a rupture of connection. It is thought that repeated and rapid returns from shame states to reconnection and attunement results in rebalancing of autonomic functioning while contributing to the gradual development of self-regulation and self-esteem.

The problem is that what began as an ancient strategy to protect our young has been conserved as the unconscious infrastructure of the later-evolving psychological processes of attachment, social status, and self-identity. The feeling of being lovable or unlovable becomes the foundation of our intimate relationships, what we think of ourselves, and how we function in groups. Those of us with core shame spend our lives with the distinct feeling that we are at risk of attack, abandonment, and even death.

The Origin of Core Shame

I don't take compliments very easily.
James Taylor

Because core shame is formed during a developmental period characterized by egocentric information processing, the loss of a parent through imprisonment, divorce, or even death is taken personally. During childhood, our parents don't leave a marriage or die from an illness; they abandon us because we weren't lovable enough for them to stay. Children can't comprehend the notion of quality time, leading them to interpret the amount of time spent together as love. If you spend most of your time away from them, they will experience it as rejection. It doesn't matter how good your excuse is or that other adults would understand; humans have been shaped to be next to and connect with their caretakers.

It appears that experiences of emotional misattunement with parents trigger the same parasympathetic reflex as being scolded and abandoned. Thus, the emotional unavailability of the parent is experienced as a rejection and interpreted as, "I'm not important, valuable, or lovable enough to be secure in my membership in the family"—which feels life threatening when your survival depends upon your family's protection. These experiences may occur in early attachment relationships when an excited expectation of connection in a child is met with inattention, indifference, or anger from a parent or caretaker. These experiences of emotional misattunement trigger the same rapid shift from sympathetic to parasympathetic control as dominance-submission displays do in other social mammals.

These ruptures of attunement and emotional connection happen between the best of parents and the healthiest of children. However, a child with a sensitive or anxious temperament may suffer greatly in the face of what appear to be normal, everyday parenting interactions. Differences in temperament and personality between parent and child can also contribute to the development of core shame because they can result in consistent misattunement.

Appropriate Versus Core Shame

> Live in such a way that you would not be ashamed to sell
> your parrot to the town gossip.
> Will Rogers

Let's clearly distinguish core shame from the appropriate kind of shame that upholds the morals and values of the group. Appropriate shame emerges slowly during childhood along with an understanding of others' expectations, an ability to judge our behaviors according to these expectations, and the control necessary to inhibit antisocial impulses. Appropriate shame supports the development of conscience, deepens our empathetic abilities, and allows us to have mutually supportive relationships.

In contrast, core shame develops in the earliest months of childhood as a reflection of how we experience our value as an individual and as a member of our family. The result of core shame is that the self is experienced as fundamentally defective, worthless, and unlovable. While being guided by appropriate shame builds positive identity, core shame results in the antithesis of self-esteem. If appropriate shame is consciously expressed as being ashamed of something you have done, core shame is a deep emotional experience of being ashamed of who and what you are. With core shame, a central part of your experience is the sense that you have lost face with no chance of redemption.

Common Consequences of Core Shame

Psychological
Depression, low self-esteem
Inappropriate self-blame
Anger, hostility, envy, and blaming others

Interpersonal
Conflict avoidance, reflective apologizing
Superficial overconfidence with reduced interpersonal
    problem solving
Intermittent rage

Biological
Decreased immunological functioning
Increased levels of cortisol and adrenaline
Decreased neuroplasticity

School and Work Performance
Maladaptive perfectionism
Reduced pride in response to success
Fear of negative evaluation and intense shame in the
    face of failure

Clients with core shame report similar themes from their childhoods. They tend to have authoritarian and critical parents or feel like they were less favored than their siblings. They are more likely to have experienced abuse, neglect, or abandonment from one or both parents or to have had parents who relied on them for emotional and practical support. Many children who have inadequate parents take on the role of being the parents' emotional caretaker from an early age.

Despite the competence of these children and their adult demeanor, the absence of adequate parenting is interpreted by their young brains as an absence of their own value. The belief is, "If I were worthy of love, my parents would have given me what I needed." At the heart of core shame is an inner certainty of being a defective person combined with the fear of this truth becoming public knowledge. Even though someone with core shame has done nothing wrong, there is also a deep sense that nothing can be done to make up for it, for the "crime" of not being loved by their parents is seldom part of their awareness.

When children with core shame are old enough to go to school, they enter the classroom anxious and fearful, anticipating academic failure and social exclusion. Because every social and educational opportunity also provides the possibility of failure, children with core shame often struggle to participate in class, interact with peers, and feel like a part of the group. Core shame is stored in implicit memory as something we never remember learning but never forget—a central aspect of the unthought known. One of the key reasons why therapy works is that we are able to uncover and name core shame and develop strategies to manage it.

Self-Esteem Versus Core Shame

Self-esteem isn't everything; it's just that there's nothing else without it.
Gloria Steinem

By the time we achieve consistent self-awareness between 5 and 10 years of age, positive self-esteem or core shame have already been programmed as social and emotional givens. It is similar in many ways to booting up your computer and being presented with a desktop that has been organized by a Microsoft or Apple operating system. You accept it as the parameters of your computing universe, unaware of the thousands of lines of programming language required to generate your reality. In other words, basic self-esteem and core shame are programmed so early in life that they are deeply known, but seldom thought about or directly articulated.

As children graduate into increasingly complex peer groups, core shame comes to shape their social world. As you might imagine, both victims and perpetrators of bullying are more likely to struggle with core shame. It becomes especially prominent during adolescence due to the heightened emphasis on being cool, acceptance into new groups, and dating. Core shame distorts social cognition and creates the experience of rejection in neutral and even positive situations. Consistent misperception of neutral interactions as rejecting creates a vicious cycle that aversively impacts victims' popularity, social status, and ability to form relationships. Their lives become marked by chronic anxiety, depression, and exhaustion from their losing struggle to achieve acceptance.

Because not knowing something can be intolerable, individuals with core shame have difficulty patiently working toward solutions. They will want quick resolutions for problems and will readily accept labels and simplistic answers from religious leaders and pop psychologists to escape the anxiety of uncertainty. Tools for regulating fear and stress will be necessary for positive change with these clients. As one of my clients put it, "I can be where I am, and I can be where I'm going, but I can't tolerate the uncertainty of being in between."

Core Shame in Psychotherapy

> *A friend is somebody who adores you even though they know the things you're most ashamed of.*
> Jodie Foster

Core shame has a number of key symptoms that therapists need to keep an eye on. Unyielding perfectionism, a lack of self-care, and choosing partners that are either abusive or nonsupportive are the most common. You also see expressions of shame in an inability to tolerate being alone or in individuals who attempt suicide after a breakup. For people with core shame, relatively minor abandonment is experienced as life threatening because it triggers implicit memories of early abandonment experiences. For some, any feedback suggesting that they are less than perfect triggers panic, making them unable to take risks, explore new ideas, or accept guidance.

When we are ashamed, our brains, like our bodies, shut down. Many who struggle with disabling shame have their cognitive and intellectual capacities negated by their negative emotions. In other words, it's hard to think rationally or to see reality clearly when your brain is telling your mind that you are in danger of abandonment and death. One of my clients described it this way: "My shame makes it impossible for me to be loved because I'm certain I'm not lovable. Therefore, if someone does love me, I can't possibly respect them because their judgment is so poor."

Establishing a positive and honest connection with clients with core shame is necessary to stimulate their brains to change. But as you can imagine, they are going to make you work very hard to earn their trust. Often, they will turn the tables on you and ask you to share your problems with them. Taking care of others is often a successful strategy to hide our own neediness from ourselves and others. Because shame leads to anger and resentment, considerable blame and hostility may be directed at you. Your dedication and availability can be experienced as a threat or attack. Clients sometimes become bullies, acting out their shame by victimizing you.

Children with parents who have problems with addictions or the law or both may have their core shame reinforced by the conscious shame of their family members. Often, children are more deeply connected to parents who mistreat them, so don't assume that abused and abandoned children don't blame themselves for what has been done to them. A kind and attentive therapist may be attacked by neglected clients because being cared for activates their sadness about the parents they never had. Clients may also direct the anger they have toward their parents at a safer target—you. Until you resolve this transference, no good deed you perform will go unpunished.

Clients with core shame can become compulsive apologizers in an attempt to avoid conflict and the anger of others, which always feels deserved. Praise bounces off them, but anything that can be interpreted as criticism will be taken hard, triggering a fight-or-flight reaction. They will overreact to interpretations because they suggest imperfection and trigger shame. Although quite intelligent, clients will avoid trying anything new unless they feel certain of success. While serving to avoid failure, it also prevents them from being open to new material, taking on challenges, and learning how to regulate their feelings of insecurity on the way to mastery. This is a reason why successful therapy correlates with a decrease in avoidance behaviors. In other words, facing our fears is a central mechanism of building new networks to inhibit fear.

Ruptures of attunement are inevitable, but a rapid return to a state of attunement supports affect regulation and contributes to the gradual development of self-regulation. It is thought that repeated and rapid returns from shame states to reconnection and attunement results in rebalancing of autonomic functioning while contributing to the gradual development of self-regulation. These repeated repairs are stored as visceral, sensory, motor, and emotional memories at all levels of the central nervous system, making the internalization of positive parenting a full-body experience. At its heart, core shame is a full-body experience of being disconnected, shunned, and expelled from social connectedness, stimulating the same brain regions activated by pain and fear. This is why Tylenol reduces the emotional impact of social rejection.

Because the level of stress associated with core shame is so high, the negative effects on brain biochemistry inhibit neuroplasticity and learning, making benefiting from therapy extremely difficult. For this reason, the transference associated with core shame is a central component of the therapy. Spanning the chasm between you and your client is the work necessary to approach and treat issues of core shame.

Therapists are just as vulnerable to core shame as clients. Clients with core shame are exceptionally good at detecting and exploiting the weaknesses and insecurities of others, especially if they fear your evaluation. Your unexplored shame, fears, and vulnerabilities may be seen and exploited by those with core shame—a good offense is a great defense. A therapist's emotional maturity and self-knowledge can make all the difference in her success. Try to discover, explore, and begin to heal some of your own brokenness before you sit across from your first client.

I'll Be Watching You

> When a woman is talking to you, listen to what she says with her eyes.
> Victor Hugo

The most important information in the world comes to us from the faces of others. Eye gaze, pupil dilation, blushing, and facial expression link us to the hearts and minds of other people. In fact, a basic preference for and recognition of faces with direct eye contact is seen during the early days of life. Later, eye gaze comes to serve as a means of social control. How many of us remember getting "the face" from a parent that made us shake in our boots? Researchers have found that while most people don't wash their hands after using a public restroom, a pair of eyes painted on the bathroom mirror will significantly increase this prosocial behavior.

The direction of eye gaze plays an especially powerful role in social communication. When we see others gazing at a person or object, looking up, or staring at something behind us, we shift our attention to share their focus. When we see a fearful or surprised look on the faces of others, we quickly reorient in the direction of their gaze to find out what they are reacting to. Increased arousal in response to eye gaze is demonstrated as early as three months of age, a process that is delayed or thwarted in people with autism spectrum disorder.

Being the object of someone else's gaze is a somewhat different story. This is one reason why eye contact can be so difficult in therapy. As the gaze of another shifts from the environment to us, our brain becomes aroused, autonomic activity increases, and the networks of the social brain go on high alert. The detection and analysis of the direct eye gaze of another is very rapid because of the significance eye contact has for physical safety and reproductive success. You can actually feel this shift as you experience yourself going on alert as someone's gaze, especially someone who looks particularly threatening or attractive, locks in on you. If people maintain eye contact for more than a few seconds, they are likely to either fight or have sex.

While direct eye gaze has the power to activate the arousal needed for a fight-flight response or a romantic approach, an averted gaze can signify rejection, ostracism, or the silent treatment. Being gazed at in an adoring way makes the gazer appear more attractive to us—most people like being adored. On the other hand, a diverted gaze from another can activate feelings of low self-esteem, decreased relational value, and the impulse to act aggressively against those who look away from us.

While our brains have been wired to orient to and gather social information via eye gaze, the language of the eyes is also influenced by early social interactions and cultural values organized in the prefrontal cortex. If we look too intently at another, it can be experienced as an insult or a sign of aggression. We monitor the gaze of our listeners to see if they are paying attention and are likely to become offended if they look away too often. In many other cultures, gaze aversion is a sign of respect to higher-ranking people and something that is expected between the sexes. Eye contact is also used to establish social dominance. Kids engage in staring contests to see who has more nerve. On the other hand, maintaining direct eye contact with a potential romantic interest can be interpreted as a sign that an approach will be accepted.

Reactions to direct eye contact can be very telling about your client's internal state. Fear or avoidance of eye contact are often symptoms of social anxiety, borderline personality disorder, and core shame. Because direct eye contact has so much meaning, looking at your clients can be experienced as anything from reassuring to threatening. How your gaze will be interpreted will be determined by an interaction between your behavior and your client's experience of you.

Sundays at the Nudist Camp

It has always been a mystery to me how men can feel themselves
honored by the humiliation of their fellow beings.
Mahatma Gandhi

There is no sweeter music to a therapist's ears than to meet a new client who desires to make radical changes by any means necessary. Jillian was such a client. Intelligent, psychologically sophisticated, but she was wracked with an array of physical illnesses that earned her the diagnosis of **conversion disorder**. She entered therapy certain that her physical suffering was a result of her childhood challenges. At 60, Jillian could see a clear trajectory from her relationship with her parents to her lifetime of emotional inhibition and ardent desire to remain invisible at all costs. Despite these challenges, she had managed to build a successful marriage, raise two healthy children, and engage in meaningful work helping victims of domestic violence.

> ### Definition: Conversion Disorder
>
> When emotions are repressed and not expressed, they set up a reverberating loop within the body that disrupts homeostatic and immunological functioning. This sets us up for what Freud called conversion disorders—a conversion of psychological and emotional pain into physical symptoms. Adding the up, left, and out model is an extension of Freud's theory with the addition of a more contemporary understanding of the underlying neurobiology. What sometimes works well with conversion is experiments in emotional expression, visibility, and assertiveness.

Both of her parents were emotionally unavailable and preoccupied with their own struggles related to self-esteem, attachment, and sexuality. Jillian's childhood was a collage of inappropriate sexualization, pathological religiosity, and keeping secrets from family and friends. She and her siblings were largely alone in coping with the chaos, confusion, and anxiety caused by their two deeply narcissistic parents. Although the story is not unusual, her need to be invisible and her core shame have a unique twist due to her parents' involvement with nudism.

At the dawn of Jillian's adolescence, her parents decided to spend each Sunday at a nudist camp. Despite her initial protests, Jillian was forced to endure long days in a wooded park being stared at by adult men. "There were no other teenagers at the camp. Other people stopped going when their kids reached adolescence, but not my parents—for us, that's when it all began." Jillian felt as if she and her sisters were being "pimped out" as a way for her parents to attract attention and make friends.

When I asked her why she went at all, she said that her mother insisted she go because there was nothing wrong with it. At the same time, she was also told never to tell anyone or her father would lose his job. Jillian's rapid submission to these wishes had been shaped by her mother's dominant and controlling nature, and she felt that rebellion was out of the question. She had been taught to follow orders and kept the secret of the Sundays at the nudist camp well into adulthood.

Jillian remembers men gathering around her family's beach chairs to stare at her and her sisters and the shame and embarrassment she felt each week. As protection against the entire experience, Jillian would bury herself in a book and try to ignore the eyes she could feel on her body. One of the after-effects of these nude Sundays was a lifelong fear of being seen or of drawing attention to herself, especially as a sexual being. She spent her life wearing the least attractive clothes she could find, shunned makeup, and downplayed anything that identified her as a woman. She looked as if she paid no attention to her clothes while in reality, her appearance was very intentional.

Her core shame and desperate need to be invisible drove her to avoid developing a career, and then to bury herself again in taking care of her children and husband. By the time I met Jillian, she had almost completely suppressed her anger, fear, and rage, and had converted them into autoimmune diseases and other physical problems. She knew that she had to learn to get these emotions out but also realized that a lifetime of hiding in fear would not change overnight.

I began my work with Jillian by doing my best to understand her core shame, fear of being seen, and the real-life struggles of staying alive. I told her that, despite her enthusiasm to forge ahead, we would need to take small steps and that she was to always stay in control of our work. This therapeutic stance is especially important with clients who have been controlled by others who have hurt them in the past.

Beginning with a focus on her medical struggles, I explained a working model that I call up, left, and out. Up, left, and out is based on the idea that our emotions are activated and stored in our bodies and need to be connected to conscious awareness by being transmitted up to the right cortical hemisphere (the apex of bodily processing), and integrated with left cortical processing in order to put words to feelings and then articulate them to ourselves and others.

While Jillian was no longer in communication with her father, her mother was compelled to keep in touch to retain her sense of control over Jillian. Jillian had coped with this by avoiding her calls as opposed to establishing a clear boundary. The first experiment was for Jillian to clearly tell her mother that she no longer wanted to communicate with her in order to establish an intentional boundary and Jillian's power.

Another way her mother influenced her life was by giving a constant stream of holiday crockery, which Jillian and her husband hated but nonetheless saved in their cupboards and closets. So the second experiment was "the breaking of the crockery," which we turned into a ritualistic destruction of her mother's influence in her life. Jillian texted me a series of pictures that depicted the piling up of shards on the garage floor. Many clients have found this exercise not only productive but also satisfying and fun.

A third experiment in visibility was to encourage Jillian to write about her work with victims of domestic violence and to organize the materials she used in her groups for possible publication. A fourth involved changing her wardrobe and appearance in the direction of being visible and even attractive to others. While all of these individual exercises may appear to be small, together they represent a gradual and manageable process to come out of the shadows and into the light.

Each of these experiments can be taken slowly, analyzed, and reconfigured for the next challenge. This allows our clients to slowly build the descending cortical circuitry necessary to inhibit amygdala activation in the face of visibility, assertiveness, and personal power. Good-enough parents help their children to accomplish this earlier in life through emotional attunement while sharing and articulating experiences. But as I've witnessed over and over again, it's never too late to learn these lessons.

CHAPTER 9

Social Status Schema: Our Place in the Social World

It is better to have a lion at the head of an army of sheep,
than a sheep at the head of an army of lions.
Daniel DeFoe

OVER THE PAST decade, many psychotherapists have adopted the concepts and discoveries that have emerged from research on human attachment. The compatibility between psychotherapy and attachment theory lies in their shared appreciation of the importance of early intimate relationships on the development and functioning of our brains, minds, and subsequent relationships. The shaping of attachment schema and an appreciation of their connection with everything from physiological regulation, to resiliency, to abstract abilities have become woven into how therapists conceptualize and work with their clients. An understanding of the connections between early attachment and the shaping and impact of core shame has also demonstrated increasing clinical utility.

What is seldom directly addressed in psychotherapy (or in the research) is the significance of social status schema, or the role played by early experience in the shaping of how we behave in social groups. Like an attachment schema, a social status schema is a form of implicit memory that shapes how we relate to others and the roles we take on in groups. In addition, social status schema leverage the primitive neural circuitry of anxiety and fear to guide us into alpha and beta roles across situations.

Knowing Your Place and Doing Your Job

As mammals became more social, larger groups came to have a competitive advantage for land, food, and other resources. But if the benefits of size are to be realized, strategies for cooperation, organization, and leadership need to be established. Social behavior within primate groups is guided by neurochemicals, hormones, and natural instincts that seem to support group survival. Despite becoming civilized, the strategies of organization and social hierarchies that are seen in our primate relatives continue largely intact within us to this day. Many of the behaviors that have been observed in monkeys, apes, and chimpanzees are readily observable on the playground, at the office, at cocktail parties, and in social media.

Although hundreds of books on attachment crowd our shelves, few even mention issues of social status. This may be because therapists are, for the most part, outside of the social arena and are involved in a solitary career. It is even a bit confusing to know where therapists fit into the social hierarchy. Another reason may be that therapists see social status as a less important spinoff of attachment security, which does not appear to be the case.

Although I can only guess as to the reasons, the avoidance of an exploration of social status schema has left a large hole in an area of vital importance to our ability to love and work. How we deal with social status is of central concern in the development of self-esteem and self-identity. This chapter and the next are an attempt to address the existence of social status schema and how we might begin to think about addressing them in psychotherapy.

Why We Have Social Status Schema

> *The manager accepts the status quo; the leader challenges it.*
> Warren Bennis

If the group is to survive, each individual has to find a role and a place within the social hierarchy that contributes to group functioning. This is how groups become a viable source of survival and the arena in which our need to love and work is expressed. The need for alphas and betas arises in the process of establishing ways to coordinate individuals within a group. Once a hierarchy is set and individual roles are established, the group can turn its focus to the business of survival. Much like ants, for whom the clarity of the roles of the queen, soldiers, and workers determine the viability of the colony, humans have to find out where they fit in, if they should lead or follow, and what their job will be.

In attachment schema, fear and anxiety are utilized to keep parents and children close to one another for safety and survival. In **social status schema**, fear and anxiety are again leveraged to keep betas respectful and in line behind alphas. Alphas gravitate to front and center positions and contain qualities that are important to direct the group. By contrast, betas focus on the alphas, look to them for leadership and guidance, and try to stay in their good graces. Similar to those with insecure attachment schema, the anxiety that drives betas to pay attention to what the alpha is doing supports group coordination, cooperation, and leadership stability. Whenever social animals form new groups, be it in the wild, the schoolyard, or the workplace, they soon begin to test each other's strength, intelligence, and resources to establish a leader.

Definition: Social Status Schema

These are constellations of biochemical interactions, instincts, and implicit memories that shape our behavior in groups. These schema determine whether we move to the front and become a leader or look to others to lead. They were organized through natural selection to enhance group coherence, coordination, and survival.

I observed a clear example of this when I witnessed a wolf's encounter with a dog on a hot Arizona afternoon. A friend who owned a wolf and I pulled onto the campus of the University of Tucson to run an errand. When the wolf jumped from the cab, a dog of about the same size ran up to him, and they immediately began to sniff and wag. Within seconds they darted from the sidewalk into a large grassy area surrounded by hedges. They both took off at full speed, and when they got to the hedge, the dog crashed out of control into the bushes while the wolf gracefully sprang over them onto the far wall.

The dog, composing itself, shot once again across the courtyard with the wolf in pursuit. In no time, the wolf was on the dog's tail. He tripped the dog by stepping on his back paw, and the dog went rolling in a cloud of dust. The dog jumped up, shook off the dust, and headed straight for us. The dog, arriving at the car behind the wolf, rolled on its back and bared its neck. In under a minute, we had witnessed a new pack establishing a dominance hierarchy. After that, they ran off to play together without any worry about who was the boss. For canines, whose social status is based on physical prowess and intelligence, the wolf had it all over the dog. Dogs have been shaped to survive by being good companions to humans, skills that hold no value in a wolf pack.

Because finding our place in the group is vital for our mutual survival, experiences of social successes and failures become imprinted in our minds, bodies, and spirits. We all seem to have a handful of victorious or humiliating memories that come to shape our self-image in groups. This imprinting shapes us into alphas or betas on our way to adulthood and maintains a powerful influence throughout life. Although they can be modified, the lingering influence of being socially shamed during childhood reflects how our brains and minds have evolved to maintain within-group social status.

Is being an alpha or a beta a matter of nature or nurture, genes, experience, personality, guts, or just a matter of circumstance? In the rest of the animal kingdom, alpha and beta parents tend to pass on their social status to their children through a combination of genes, biology, and behaviors. On the surface, humans are a bit more complex, judging each other on a wide array of attributes including size and strength, attractiveness, wealth, how we dress, and being cool. And unlike other animals, we spend our lives participating in a number of groups across which our status may vary. While social status cannot be reduced to simplistic distinctions between alphas and betas, the personalities and internal experiences of individuals that fit each category can be helpful in therapy.

Of Alphas and Betas

> *Innovation distinguishes between a leader and a follower.*
>
> Steve Jobs

Alphas are the hub of the social wheel, the ones that others look to in times of anxiety and uncertainty for protection and guidance. In a herd of elephants, the alpha is most likely to be the oldest female, the matriarch, who has the accumulated knowledge of the locations of water holes and the ins and outs of child rearing. In a troop of gorillas, the alpha is usually the largest male, the silverback. The silverback is best equipped to protect the troop from attack and more likely to father larger male children who will do the same. Thus, the alpha isn't determined strictly by size, gender, or fighting power but by the value of that individual to the survival of the group in a particular environment.

One way to think of the alpha is as the brain of the group that organizes group behavior in a way to optimize group survival. The successful group is the one with the most effective leadership matched to the survival challenges, be it strength, cunning, or forethought. Predicting and adapting to the ever-emerging present is the prime directive of the human brain and the group. I emphasize the diversity of what it means to be an alpha because of our cultural bias to equate alpha status with a particular gender, body type, or set of behaviors. Social status is all about adaptation to particular ecosystems.

As I mentioned earlier, social schema, like attachment

schema, are programmed at multiple levels, including the bio-chemistry and neuroanatomy of our brains. Even before birth, our mothers' experiences, emotions, and states of mind begin influencing the production and availability of neurochemicals in our nervous system. At the same time, the neural networks that determine our dispositions and relationships begin to take shape. And while this shaping process continues throughout life, early experiences are usually the most influential.

Relationships with parents and siblings and early peer interactions appear to be of central importance. Most children start out seeing their parents as alphas—a view that establishes competition with parents as part of normal development. Simultaneously, children depend on their parents' love and benevolence for survival. Emotionally mature parents see their children as separate people, encouraging their development and success by modulating their competitive urges in ways that allow their children to feel successful and to build confidence.

If parents didn't receive the parenting and security they needed as children, their unresolved issues may become part of the childhood drama of the next generation. Emotionally immature parents may not be able to remember to be parents in situations of competition, giving their children repeated experiences of failure and shame. These parents will see their children as threats, and they will not be able to express encouragement or pride in their child's accomplishments. Dominant, insecure parents may micromanage their children and undermine their children's emerging confidence and skill development. Parents may also unconsciously pass the disappointment they felt from their parents onto their own children.

Sons of very successful fathers have a particular challenge: "How do I measure up?" Successful fathers are often far more appreciated at work than they are at home. Many fathers who are self-made and work hard to provide for their children come to resent their children for not sharing their initiative and work ethic. They often forget that their motivations were born of the same deprivation, fear, and struggle from which they have shielded their children. It is very easy to be successful and create children that you can't relate to, which may be why so many of the men I've worked with feel that their fathers were disappointed in them.

Loss of a parent by death or abandonment generally leaves children in a compromised position. For some children, being abandoned is demoralizing, and it deprives them of a guide into adulthood. For others, the absent parent triggers a fighting spirit that inspires their power and success. I suspect that, regardless of the outcome, parental loss creates a deep sense of insecurity that is compensated for either by a drive to succeed or by a loss of motivation. Part of being an alpha or beta is modeling the social behaviors of your parents. The absence of the parent may, by definition, be a detriment to a child's establishment of a place in the group.

The most obvious field of social dominance is physical and emotional aggression, what we call bullying. Children who are different in some way are more likely to be bullied; they are easily identifiable targets, often suffer from low self-esteem, have difficulty defending themselves, and are less likely to be defended by others. Being victimized by bullies can have serious emotional and behavioral consequences, especially if the abuse is severe and/or chronic. These painful experiences at vulnerable developmental stages can have lifelong effects. Never underestimate the impact of childhood bullying on the brains, minds, and hearts of your clients.

Most incidents of bullying are public displays, witnessed and remembered by others in the service of establishing or maintaining a social hierarchy. The public nature of being bullied enhances the amount of shame experienced by the victim, which increases the bully's social status (at least in his own eyes). The feelings of shame associated with being publicly bullied reaffirm beta status both within victims and in the eyes of others.

Some individuals are able to translate experiences of being bullied into rage that they use to subsequently challenge and defeat the alpha. On the other hand, a large number of adults who experienced chronic bullying during childhood and adolescence continue to experience symptoms of their victimization in adulthood. Adult betas usually remember incidents of being bullied and hold onto it as evidence of their lower social status. Reports of depression, anxiety, blunted emotions, sleep disturbance, and symptoms of PTSD are common. What we label as psychiatric symptoms, when viewed through another lens, serve as lifelong mechanisms of social control.

The Four Schema

> My attitude is never to be satisfied, never enough, never.
> Duke Ellington

The group, like each individual brain, is an organ of adaptation in service of survival that depends on the complementarity of alphas and betas to support group survival. Groups usually contain a few alphas and many betas. As groups form, members jockey for position, display their abilities, and strive to develop alliances. On the surface, this behavior looks like it is driven by self-interest. Looking at it from a distance reveals that all the social climbing, challenges, rough-and-tumble play, and aggression also serve to provide the group with a pool of potential leaders. And while we generally associate alpha-beta conflict with males, it is equally important among females and occurs to different degrees across genders.

I have observed at least four social status groups in my personal and professional relationships. There are two groups of individuals who are well matched to their social status, whom I call natural alphas and natural betas. A third group consists of those who know they are betas, but aspire to become alphas (aspirational alphas), and a fourth group who think they are alphas, but are actually betas (pseudoalphas). Both aspirational alphas and pseudoalphas can be considered insecure because there is a conflict between their desired social status and the programming of their biochemistry, thought patterns, and behaviors.

A very small number of people are natural alphas—those who are good at and derive satisfaction from being leaders. While not deaf to the opinions of others, natural alphas pay less attention to group opinion, focusing on their instincts and inner vision to guide them. Natural alphas always have an eye on the future, and their dissatisfaction with the status quo is a secret source of pleasure. These qualities of the natural alpha provide the group with imagination, vision, and expanded adaptational capacities. Natural alphas don't have to try to be alphas; their status comes from an inner sense of security, the anticipation and even expectation of success, and a goodness of fit with their natural wiring.

Another large group of people are natural betas and are well matched to this status. Natural betas are not haunted by fears of underachieving or keeping their light under a bushel. They enjoy their jobs and social relationships, and they are satisfied with what they have achieved. Natural betas are fine with external structure and generally feel most confident and happy when there are external rules and plans to follow. They tend to focus on the present situation and make the best of the resources at hand. It is easy to see how a large number of natural betas would be vital to a successful empire.

The Four Social Status Schema

Natural Alphas: Natural leaders who feel confident and free to have a voice in the group and lead when necessary. They are biologically programmed to be less anxious, more exploratory, and more resilient to physical and social stress.

Natural Betas: Natural followers who gain meaning and satisfaction in contributing to the group by fulfilling an established role. They are biologically programmed to be somewhat more anxious and more influenced by the opinions of others.

Aspirational Alphas: Biologically and psychologically programmed to be betas, these individuals have the desire and often the ability to take on an alpha role. Their desire to be seen and express themselves comes into conflict with their programming to be part of the group and follow the leader. These are the individuals who most often seek therapy and career coaching for assistance with personal growth.

Pseudoalphas: Individuals with the outward persona of an alpha but the internal conflicts of a beta. Pseudoalphas think of themselves as alphas and suppress their anxieties and insecurities through denial, bullying others, and bravado. Pseudoalphas are usually sent to therapy by others who find them difficult to live and work with or because of substance abuse or other self-damaging behaviors.

Neither natural alphas nor natural betas experience status conflict because their brains, minds, and relationships are aligned. If a natural beta is accused of having a fear of failure or a natural alpha is called a narcissist, it's quickly shrugged off—nothing breeds confidence like knowing who you are and where you fit in your tribe. The optimum group might contain a natural alpha, many natural betas, and a few aspirational alphas to be ready when leadership roles become available.

Aspirational alphas feel like betas but suspect that they may have what it takes to be alphas and possess the drive to pursue leadership roles. While their minds tell them to be visible, take risks, and take charge, their brains are conditioned to follow the leader. Thus, aspirational alphas are in conflict—on the one hand champing at the bit to be seen, while on the other, ambivalent about making their ideas and intentions public. Aspirational alphas live in a dynamic tension between the drive to express themselves and their fear of visibility. This manifests as self-doubt (Am I smart and strong enough to make it?) and shame (Am I worthy of the love and admiration of others?).

Then, there are those who have attained the appearance of alpha status, yet are wired like betas. Although I'm not sure this group exists in other animals, it certainly does among humans. These individuals, whom I refer to as pseudoalphas, are often highly successful executives, doctors, attorneys, and politicians who function at a high level and have the respect and admiration of their group. Except for those few people who know them best, most see these people as natural alphas. However, pseudoalphas experience the greatest anxiety, insecurity, and conflict of all because they live in constant fear of being exposed. They are often ineffectual or toxic leaders whose narcissistic defenses and insecurities become group liabilities.

For natural alphas and betas, brains, minds, and relationships are aligned, which results in happiness, success, and minimal conflict. For aspirational and pseudoalphas, their brains, minds, and relationships are unaligned, which results in psychological and social conflict, creating a variety of behaviors that betray their inner struggles. Overall, these insecure betas are dissatisfied with their lives. They are frustrated and angry with others; they don't perform up to their potential, and they usually feel disappointed in themselves. These are clients who come to therapy for help.

The Brains and Minds of Alphas and Betas

> *Mastering others is strength. Mastering yourself is true power.*
> Lao Tzu

The brains and minds of alphas are best characterized as being less fearful and anxious, more resilient to stress, and oriented toward exploration and creativity. On a biological level, human alphas are therefore less afraid to take risks or experience failure, and are more willing to try again after failure. Their memory circuitry is wired in a way that leads them to have positive expectations for the future and to anticipate positive outcomes. In other words, optimism is central to their experience. Psychologically, alphas feel free to give voice to their opinion and are not preoccupied with how others perceive them. They feel comfortable being visible, and they don't mind being the center of attention. Alphas also feel confident in plotting a course of action for themselves and others, and they are willing to accept the consequences of their decisions. All of these attributes would support successful group leadership in the vast majority of survival situations. Although many of these attributes parallel aspects of secure attachment, most securely attached individuals are not programmed to be alphas.

Alpha Wiring Shapes Us Into Leaders

Bodily Reactions	A resting state that can respond to threat when it arises Preparedness to act if necessary
Emotions	Calm, curious, enthusiastic, optimistic
Thoughts	Expectations of positive outcomes Minimal concern about potential failures Accurate assessment of external situations Accurate assessment of personal strengths, weaknesses, and abilities
Behaviors	Exploratory, risk taking Prepared to solve problems

Betas experience their social and inner worlds quite differently. Betas are more anxious, concerned about how others view them, and fear failure. Being visible, singled out, and not deferring to others is experienced as a threat. Being seen at first triggers fear, and then a parasympathetic reaction resulting in retreat and deflation. Betas feel far more comfortable blending in with the group and following the leader. They may experience panic attacks when they do public speaking or gain social visibility. They experience relief when they don't have to make decisions or are passed over when it's time to make a toast.

The brains of betas are wired in ways that result in greater vigilance for environmental dangers, most notably, what they see in the eyes of others. Eyes have a direct line to the amygdala and signal other people's opinion of who we are and what we are doing. Thus, the eyes of others signal betas about what to do and whether the alpha is pleased with them. In the absence of an alpha, betas have an inner set of eyes along with an inner voice that keeps them in line—what Freud called superego. Betas' insecurity about their abilities and status amplifies the alpha's power. Betas' role in evolution was to be docile, agreeable, and controllable through intimidation, both by others and by the inner voices that keep them in line even when no one is watching.

Beta Wiring Shapes Us Into Followers

Bodily Reactions	Hypervigilance for threat
	Submission response
Emotions	Anxiety, fear, sadness, depression, demoralization
Thoughts	Experience of danger, inferiority, anticipation of failure
	Expectation of being shamed, feeling fraudulent
Behaviors	Avoidance of situations associated with anxiety
	Hiding, invisibility, social withdrawal, avoiding risks
	Underselling skills and abilities
	Avoiding situations where failure is possible

The attributes of alphas and betas support group coherence and coordination through their complementarity: one group provides leaders, and the other provides good soldiers. The shaping of alphas and betas allows them to link together into a group mind that allows the group to function as a unit. Alphas seek solutions to problems while betas wait for the signal to act. The brains of alphas and betas have been shaped to link together in the service of the group. And while all of us experience our social status as an individual accomplishment or failure, the fact that we have a status and role surreptitiously serves the survival of the group.

Changing Our Status Schema

> *A woman without a man is like a fish without a bicycle.*
>
> Irina Dunn

On the surface, our culture tells us we are all capable of being alphas—anyone can become rich, become famous, or be president. Because it only happens for a relative few, the vast majority of us are at risk of feeling like failures. Given that most of us are wired to be betas, conflict between our programming often arises. The social mandate to be an alpha collides with our unconscious programming to get in line and not make trouble. But what if you have what it takes to be an alpha, but your brain and mind have beta programming that stems from core shame?

The goal of therapy, counseling, and coaching is to help those we work with to gain security by aligning their brains, minds, and relationships. Natural alphas and betas are not going to come for help about their social status schema. Rather, mostly aspirational alphas and an occasional pseudoalpha will find their way to us. The message to these folks is that if you have been programmed to be a beta, there are ways to learn how to be an alpha. This is accomplished by using our minds to develop strategies and learn new skills. It takes time, work, and the ability to face our fears. It also takes a guide, or a therapist, to help us along on our journey.

For many clients, moving from beta to alpha status is the central focus of psychotherapy. Many people that come to therapy are either aspirational alphas who want help achieving their dreams or pseudoalphas whose lives have been negatively impacted by the incongruity of their inner and outer worlds. One of the most common problems in our clients is that they have lived their entire lives evaluating themselves based on how others see them, and they have never learned to have their own feelings and perspectives. If this sounds like a form of brainwashing and social control, it is. Not by a cult leader, but by an evolutionary strategy shaped over millions of years.

Aspirational alphas will experience success that leads them to public speaking, which will trigger anxiety and even panic attacks. They have difficulty being assertive in situations that require it, or they have a hard time confronting people when difficult emotions are involved. Aspirational alphas may have difficulty telling their employees what to do even though that is part of their job. It will be hard for them to be self-promoting, so they will watch others who are less capable and less experienced get promoted over them. Outside of work they may habitually let others go ahead of them in line, have the good table at the restaurant, or step aside and let someone else ask the more desirable woman on a date.

These are all beta behaviors that, if engaged in from time to time, are not a cause for concern. However, if they represent a lifestyle and if the thought of doing otherwise triggers notable anxiety, these behaviors most likely reflect beta programming that will keep clients from moving forward in their lives. Sometimes people who are wired as betas will create or adopt philosophical and religious beliefs that justify their beta behavior—turn the other cheek, be without ego, take care of everyone else before yourself. And while these are wonderful philosophies, consider the possibility that they relieve betas from facing their fears of being visible.

Social Status in Psychotherapy

> *Go confidently in the direction of your dreams!*
> *Live the life you've imagined.*
> Henry David Thoreau

The central component in any helping relationship is the establishment of a safe and trusting connection. The warmth, acceptance, and positive regard that are characteristics of successful therapists, coaches, teachers, and parents are the opposite of fighting for social dominance. This is not a coincidence—helping and healing relationships have been shaped by our need to activate neural networks related to adaptation, learning, and growth. The need to be in therapy and the need to become a therapist are driven by our deep desire to be seen, feel felt, and to connect with others.

It is always important to keep in mind that each therapeutic relationship has at least two narratives going on at the same time. First is the surface narrative, or the interaction between a warm, supportive therapist and a client who is open to being helped. But the narrative below the surface, the process narrative, is a reenactment of the social status struggles and attachment histories of each individual. Therapist and client come into the consulting room with their own histories that get played out as part of the therapeutic relationship—transference and countertransference. Ignore this level of the relationship and progress may be negated by the activation of primal power dynamics.

From the beginning, one of the great drives of psychotherapy was to forward the process of conscious evolution. The problem with an exclusive focus on this goal in therapy is that we are still primates that retain many of our primitive mammalian sensibilities. We compete for status and the best mates in the same way as other animals. When client and therapist enter the consultation room, they are also animals in competition for survival.

As you will see in Chapter 10, assisting someone on the path to alpha status is different than traditional models of psychotherapy. It is more interactive and outward facing and requires the therapist to also play the role of parent, cheerleader, and sometimes a tough opponent. It involves more of the masculine aspects of reparenting than the maternal qualities that we usually strive for.

Helping Clients Become Alphas

If you want a quality, act as if you already had it.
—William James

OF THE FOUR social status categories, it is the aspirational alpha that is most likely to seek our help. Aspirational alphas long to be recognized for their skills and abilities, to play with the big kids, and to have their ideas taken seriously. While aspiring to be an alpha doesn't ensure success, many of our clients are driven to give it a try. This drive, shaped by natural selection to provide challenges to present leadership, should be respected and encouraged. This striving, older than the human race, is at the core of the myth of the hero. It is the journey that many of us face to overcome external obstacles and inner doubt to win the prizes of adulthood: riches, love, and freedom.

Can a beta become an alpha? "Why not?" We know we can change our minds, and we know that our brains remain plastic throughout life. So why couldn't a beta earn alpha status? If the core of beta status is a group of bodily reactions, feelings, thoughts, and behaviors, why can't our clients rewire their brains for alpha status? While it might sound like a superficial cliché, "fake it till you make it" is a form of imitation, which is central to how humans evolved to learn. This is why we expend so much energy at play early in life—to practice skills in a safe environment that we will someday need in the real world. We play house, we play war, and we play doctor long before any of these situations become real. For a beta to become an alpha, our clients have to create a set of goals and a plan to get there. Consider the following three general steps.

First, work with your clients to cocreate an image of what they want to become. Explore their vision of life and create a list of alpha attributes in line with their goals. Support them to behave, think, and feel in ways that are in line with their goals. Prepare your clients with the awareness that although "alphaness" will feel alien at first, continual practice will make it eventually come to feel like a part of the self. This is not a trick—imitation has been woven into our brains as a key way to learn and is linked directly to our imaginations. The natural flow is from imitation to improvisation to invention.

Second, because a large part of our self-identity is reflected in the stories we tell about ourselves, help clients examine their self-stories for unconscious beta programming. As therapists, we can help clients examine their stories, replacing beta thoughts, emotions, and behaviors with those of alphas. Are their self-stories blueprints for exploration, leadership, and courage? Or are they full of compromises, excuses, and waiting to be saved by an alpha? Aspiring alphas need to realize that stories can contain and perpetuate underestimations of their abilities. They also need to know that their life stories can be rewritten with new plots, trajectories, and conclusions.

Third, in the face of fear, beta programming activates the parasympathetic nervous system, signaling us to shrink and withdraw. If you are scheduled to give a presentation, it will activate anticipatory anxiety, activate negative thoughts in your head, and even trigger panic attacks as you approach the podium. These beta strategies are stored in our amygdala and are designed to keep us following the leader. So work to have your clients reframe anxiety and fear from an alarm to retreat into a signal to advance. One of the strongest correlates of therapeutic success is the reduction of avoidance reactions. Approaching fears provides the opportunity to rewire primitive fear circuitry from a beta to alpha bias. A key difference between alpha and beta status is our reaction to challenge and the unknown; betas retreat while alphas advance. Courage is not the absence of fear, but moving forward in spite of fear. Courage is required for the aspirational alpha to gain alpha status.

The Alpha Shift

> *Only one thing matters, one thing: to be able to dare!*
> Fyodor Dostoyevsky

Aspiring to be an alpha is a big challenge, especially if our clients' beta status is leveraged by core shame. This requires us to be both supportive and challenging in a balance appropriate to each client's current needs. We have to both empathize with their fears and encourage them to face their demons. You can act as a guide to addressing their shame, changing their minds, and taking control of their lives.

What follow are some contrasting characteristics of alphas and betas. Each of these differences can be converted into strategies to combat beta programming and core shame. Have them start by choosing one of these alpha ways of being and live it to the best of their ability. Sessions should include the creation of experiments in alpha style, recaps of last week's experiments, and problem solving when roadblocks arise. As clients reach a level of proficiency with one alpha characteristic, they can adopt another and repeat the process.

The mind of an insecure beta distorts information in the service of keeping him or her in a submissive posture. As you teach your clients to check their thoughts for negative distortions, they will learn to listen less to the negative information provided by their beta programming. You will soon notice that the strategies of becoming an alpha map almost exactly onto the goals of most forms of psychotherapy, executive coaching, and parental guidance—no coincidence there. Many emotional and interpersonal struggles are driven by the underlying and unspoken struggle with the beta programming within our social status schema.

#1 Alphas Are Confident

> *With confidence you have won even before you have started.*
> Marcus Garvey

Alphas' security in their abilities is their best ally. They are willing to take risks based on their own judgment and are open to correction and modification to improve their strategies. When they are wrong in their interactions with others, they apologize. Their apologies are not about who they are, but for something they have done wrong. In contrast, insecure betas often reflexively apologize for doing something whether or not it is their fault. Beneath the surface, the apologies are not about what they've done, but are a social signal of submission.

Betas reflexively apologize because they feel like they are always on probation—a good description of core shame. Alternatively, pseudoalphas with big egos blame others for failure and are constantly proving themselves by stating their qualifications, connections, and pedigrees—they are the ones with all the extra letters after their names. They are the first to correct others and to display condescending attitudes. Pseudoalphas' bigger egos are a handicap because they are too sensitive and insecure regarding the opinions of others.

#2 Alphas Take Responsibility for Outcomes

> *The price of greatness is responsibility.*
> Winston Churchill

Alphas take responsibility for their behaviors and the success of the group; betas make excuses for failure and blame others. When failures do occur, the alpha sees an opportunity to make changes and is flexible enough to devise alternative plans that decrease the probability of failure. Alphas attempt to control contingencies necessary to succeed, and they use failure as a learning experience for the next time. With this strategy, they succeed more often and have greater confidence in their eventual success. Because insecure betas anticipate failure, they spend significant amounts of energy preparing excuses and making lists of others who have thwarted their progress and external factors that caused them to fail. This prevents betas from having to address their own failings, a short-term solution that keeps their core shame at bay.

If you find clients making excuses for their failures and shortcomings, you can interrupt the cycle by helping them to expand their sense of personal responsibility. Have them ask themselves, "What could I have done differently?" imagining a "do over" with better information and a different strategy. You can help clients figure out how they can learn from whatever challenge they are facing. To change our status, we all need to take personal responsibility in any way we can. This will change how we view ourselves as well as how others perceive us.

#3 Alphas Don't Fear Failure

> Never, never, never give up.
> Winston Churchill

Alphas are fascinated by obstacles and see them as opportunities to expand their problem-solving abilities. While alphas see failures as prerequisites for success, betas fixate on failure and revisit it in their minds on a regular basis. This keeps betas in a submissive posture, looking to the alpha for guidance. For betas with core shame, failures are traumatic referendums on their value as human beings, so the possibility of failure makes them avoid taking on challenges. If living life was driving a car, betas would steer using the rearview mirror, fixating on past failures. Alphas hold onto the wheel, watching the road ahead. Alphas play to win, not to avoid losing.

Have your clients reframe failures as a list of lessons to be learned and commit to learning the lessons of therapy. Instead of avoiding our weaknesses, we need to work on each one in turn until they become strengths.

#4 Alphas Keep Their Own Council

> A man who wants to lead an orchestra must turn his back on the crowd.
> James Cook

A natural alpha is less influenced by peer pressure and group-think. Alphas think of and promote new ideas to offer the tribe new options. Related to this is the alpha's use of inner values to guide thinking. While not at the mercy of the perception of others, they are also not blind to it. Alphas value other people's opinions as data and potential sources of valuable information. They can be hurt by criticism, but this is not automatic. They first think about the feedback to see if it aligns with their own experience; they consider the source and then cull out the valuable information.

Clients on the way to alpha status should not waste time worrying about what others think of them. On the other hand, they need to pay attention to the political aspects of a situation. The difference is, it's not personal; for alphas, it's about supporting teams, building culture, and reaching the goal. As soon as it becomes personal, anxiety rises and executive functioning plummets. When insecure betas are criticized, that criticism goes down a tube into their stomachs, and they feel forced to take it in. Instead, have your clients imagine putting the criticism on a tray, taking a look, and considering whether they want to swallow it or not. Remember, very few people are actually paying attention to us—betas are worried about what you think of them, and alphas have better things to do. The judgment is inside our own heads; do not let clients be fooled into thinking that it comes from others.

#5 Alphas Are Able to Regulate Their Emotions

> You must be the person you have never had the courage to be.
> Paulo Coelho

Alphas don't have tantrums. Explosive and uncontrolled expressions of emotion come from feelings of frustration, helplessness, and fear. People who scream at their employees, beat their spouses and children, or lose control of themselves are seldom alphas. This doesn't mean that alphas don't lose it from time to time. The difference is that these are exceptions to their usual behaviors. Pseudoalphas misinterpret aggression as power—it is actually the opposite. Someone stalking a partner who left him or her demonstrates vulnerability and desperation—not power.

If clients have a tendency to become wound up and anxious, teach them to pay attention to and gain control of their breathing. Because our breath is synchronized with our autonomic nervous system and bodily arousal, awareness and control of our breath is a way to keep our bodies and emotions regulated, a good tool to have in anxiety-provoking situations. Breathing and talking go hand in hand; while clients are learning to be aware of their breath, they should also pay attention to the pace and tone of their voice. Remember that the speed, tone, and pitch of our voices will influence our self-perceptions and the perceptions of others. A slower, softer, firmer voice can be used to great effect. If you find clients darting from place to place, you can remind them that alphas feel comfortable in their bodies and own the space they move through. We all get anxious; being an alpha and overcoming core shame means that we are in control, not the anxiety.

#6 Alphas Have Goals and a Plan to Get There

> Leadership is the capacity to translate vision into reality.
> Warren Bennis

Typically, alphas have a vision of the future in mind, focusing on what is best for the group. Their brains and minds are shaped to think beyond the present and beyond the information given. This is why, at least in the modern world, alphas so often have careers while betas have jobs. The alpha is a hard worker with a purpose who doesn't expect to succeed through the efforts of others. Alphas know that nothing great is accomplished without a combination of vision and hard work, and they put in consistent time and energy toward reaching their goals.

Betas are shaped to rely on the structure provided by others. In contrast, even when working for others, alphas see themselves as the CEO of their own careers. They are doing a good job in the present and have an eye toward an imagined future. For alphas, the ideal future continues to offer challenges in line with their expanding knowledge and abilities. This ties in with the fact that tribes always need a leader thinking outside the box in case the current situation changes—a good definition of adaptation.

Some clients may not think beyond the given situation; however, you can structure a set of exercises and questions to remind clients to pay attention to these issues, creating a prosthetic executive system through a set of tasks and questions. Encourage clients to challenge their ideas and beliefs instead of maintaining maladaptive patterns. From an outsider's perspective, you can help clients examine new paths and ideas.

#7 Alphas Understand and Utilize the Power of Words

> Better than a thousand hollow words, is one word that brings peace.
> Buddha

Storytelling has been the primary mechanism of teaching and guiding group behavior for most of human history. Alphas know how to tell a good story and are capable of using humor and self-disclosure to communicate their points. True alphas are aware of the power of their words, so they measure them carefully and to their advantage. The loudest person in the room, the one who won't let you get a word in edgewise, or the one that talks while you are talking is always a pseudoalpha. Alphas know how to listen to others, and, more importantly, to themselves.

Learning to be still, listen, and carefully consider what others are saying is a central component of mindful awareness. This is an important lesson for clients and therapists. Compulsive talking is almost always an indication of anxiety that keeps us from connecting with others and in exile from ourselves. We need to learn not to speak reflexively. This takes practice. By allowing ourselves time to think and consider the impact of our words, we can become more self-aware while becoming more effective in our interactions with others. The shift from beta to alpha status includes learning to listen better and to talk less while saying more.

#8 *Alphas Accept Their Vulnerability*

> *Perfection itself is imperfection.*
> Vladimir Horowitz

Alphas are less afraid to face their faults and are therefore better able to overcome their failures. Alphas know they are flawed, so they give way to the leadership of others in areas of weakness and affiliate with others who have the skills and abilities they need to succeed. Because insecure betas try to be perfect, they constantly experience falling short, which then makes them more insecure. Betas always feel like victims of an internal blackmail—they don't want the secret of their imperfection to get out.

While betas are too afraid to admit their faults or mistakes, alphas experience the freedom of vulnerability. By outing themselves as imperfect, they avoid being blackmailed by the inner voices of shame. As a therapist, you can encourage your beta clients to look at and accept their flaws and integrate them into their self-image. By creating a safe environment, clients will be able explore their imperfections without being overwhelmed by fear or anxiety. Once clients accomplish a deep realization that they do not have to be perfect, they can view their faults more objectively and learn how much power lies in being human.

#9 Alphas Select Their Partners Consciously

> *Happy is the man who finds a true friend . . . in his wife.*
> Franz Schubert

In both work and personal relationships, betas tend to be attracted to others who are attracted to them. They skip over assessing the value of the person or their goodness of fit for a relationship. Because of this, insecure betas with core shame often find themselves in relationships that don't live up to their expectations. To make matters worse, they project their inadequacies onto their partners and blame them for their disappointments. Still other betas choose partners who possess the qualities they crave for themselves but come to resent them later for these same characteristics.

Alphas select their partners consciously; that is, they listen to both their hearts and their heads. The challenge for alphas is not to find a partner who is attracted to them, but to find someone who is comfortable with their strength and abilities.

Alphas know that it is important for them to find partners both in work and their personal lives who won't be threatened by who they are—another secure alpha or beta. In considering what they would like in a relationship, the decide whether they would like the complementarity of a beta or the partnership of another alpha. Different situations will require different kinds of partnerships, and the alpha is mindful of these issues.

#10 Alphas Are Not Afraid to Be Quiet or Alone

> *Loneliness is the poverty of the self; solitude is the richness of the self.*
> May Sarton

Being alone with one's thoughts should be a source of strength, not terror. Betas don't feel it is up to them to make a decision about their own worth, so they are obsessed with how they look to others. Betas give others the power to judge their value as human beings. They struggle to get the attention of others in any way possible, relying on affirmation from others and seeing themselves as they imagine others see them. Alphas have the capacity to be alone and can draw strength and greater perspective from their inner resources.

As your clients learn to challenge their negative internal voices, they will also learn to care less about the opinions of others and find their inner world to be a safer place, a place where they can choose what to think, how to feel, and make decisions about their lives. Remind clients that the dialogue in their head can be changed—it is just another set of learned behaviors. If they can become strong enough to care for and protect the child within them, they will also learn that they can be good company to themselves.

Terapia Con Cojones

> *I am the greatest. I said that even before I knew I was.*
> Muhammad Ali

So how can therapy address core shame and guide the process of earning alpha status? Half of the answer lies in what we already do—focusing on empathy, understanding, and relationship building. The other half is something that therapists often avoid: challenging our clients to toughen up, take bigger risks, and face off with their demons.

Beta status programming is stored and organized in the brain in the same neural networks and in similar manner to traumatic experiences. The primitive amygdala executive system is doing its best to protect us from whatever it pairs with danger. This is how the beta brain pairs confidence, anger, and assertiveness with social anxiety, danger, and fear. The problem is that when we abdicate our anger, we also surrender our power and ability to be seen by others, rendering us betas looking for guidance.

Therapists have two weapons against this beta conditioning. The first is our ability to be amygdala whisperers and gradually teach our clients how to soothe their fears. Second, we can help clients get in touch with their primitive anger and rage, the only instinct that is more powerful than fear. The first part is very common in psychotherapy; it is a strongly feminine profession. More women become therapists and more women come to therapy as clients. The second step is far less common. People who become therapists often avoid their own anger and are afraid of it in their clients. This internally motivated avoidance of anger is supported by the realistic fear that female therapists have in response to activating the rage of male clients when they are alone together. All understandable.

In the same way that women can't father boys, female therapists have an understandably difficult time helping male clients deal with their anger. Be it different ways of relating, a desire for connection, or just fear of physical violence, female therapists shy away from angry feelings men have in their struggle to be alphas. Instead, female therapists tend to go after the sadness. The sadness is extremely important and should not be overlooked. However, men need to get enraged, give the hairy eyeball, and go on the warpath. Women generally want no part of this. On the other hand, female therapists will only be able to help their female clients to get in touch with their anger, assertiveness, and power to the degree to which they are in touch with their own.

Machine Gun Kelly

Anybody can become angry—that is easy. But to be angry with the right person . . . for the right purpose, in the right way—that is not easy.
Aristotle

An exercise that I call Machine Gun Kelly may be helpful for clients and therapists who need to access their anger. The first step consists of imagining the frightening alpha—often the father, an abusive teacher, or an abusive spouse that your client may be terrified to stand up to. The exercise is to imagine a scene where the client remembers being terrified and frightened. This doesn't necessarily mean that the frightening alpha was physically threatening. It could also mean that the alpha looked at your client with disgust, rejection, or just turned his or her back. The important element is that your client's brain recorded this as an interaction that was threatening to his or her survival.

The next step is to encourage your client to grab a machine gun and open fire. Get into imagining it—cut them up, watch the pieces fly; if you want to get into it at a deeper level, it's okay to go a little further; clients can use martial arts–type yells and gestures to help get the emotions out. Instruct your client to cut the frightening alpha to ribbons. Then, discuss the client's feelings, which may range from exhilaration to fear to sympathy for the alpha. (Such an extreme imaginary scenario will push repressed clients to either experience or resist the assignment. Many times, just discussing their unwillingness to engage in the visualization will lead to considerable exploration, understanding, and growth.)

After they have expressed their feelings, have clients imagine putting the frightening alpha back together and do it again. Try and add something different each time so as not to make it a routine or stereotyped set of behaviors without feelings. All reactions are welcome and open for discussion and interpretation. Use your judgment to assist clients in expressing their anger in whatever way makes sense given their history, challenges, and personality. The important thing is that you help your clients find a way to channel their anger outward in an assertive and powerful way. (Keep in mind that the machine gun is optional. Reshaping the assignment into running over the frightening alpha's prized possession or spray painting his or her house may be enough of a challenge for many clients.)

What most clients notice after multiple imaginings is (1) that it becomes easier, (2) that emotions shift from fear to anger to rage, and (3) eventually it becomes boring. You are shooting—no pun intended—for boring. As the fear is processed and the power dynamics shift, the image eventually loses its effectiveness. As the fear memories are integrated with current cortical processing, there will be a shift in how the client thinks and feels about the threatening alpha. This doesn't always work—but it's worth a try. At the very least, you will gather some very interesting information about your client's inner world and how deep the early alpha-beta status is imprinted into the client's central nervous system. (*Caution*—do not use this exercise with those who have trouble controlling their anger, but only with those who have a lifelong pattern of difficulty being in touch with and expressing their anger.)

At first, most clients will push back at this exercise from a combination of fear and loyalty to the alpha—a loyalty that is driven by our primitive instincts. The same underlying instinct most likely drives Stockholm syndrome, where captives begin to align with and feel sympathetic toward their captors. As with all primitive reflexes, if they go too far, they result in nonfunctional and symptomatic behavior. Foraging can become hoarding; a desire for order turns into obsessive-compulsive disorder, and the need to be a good boy or girl can lead us to abdicate our opinions, beliefs, and instincts for self-preservation.

Rage Against the Machine

Education is indoctrination if you're white—subjugation if you are black.
James Baldwin

Rage is an extreme expression of the fight-flight response triggered by a threat to a loved one or an offense against something we hold dear. Rage correlates with surges of adrenaline that lead us to be able to do things we wouldn't ordinarily be able to. Time slows; our attention becomes razor sharp, and rational thought is temporarily suspended. Although rage is usually seen as counterproductive, it can also serve us. We have all heard stories of the extraordinary strength exhibited by a parent to protect or save a child. Rage can also be used to our own advantage against unconscious programming. The primitive power of rage has the ability to counteract the fear that locks us into being betas.

Betas often have rage when they are overwhelmed by frustration and feelings of powerlessness. This impotent rage is taken out on those closest to them because they feel safe enough to express it. We know that the presence of the alpha will decrease both the testosterone levels and the aggression of betas in groups. When this prohibition created by the presence of the alpha is removed, rage is taken out on the most vulnerable—children, animals, partners, or whoever will or has to tolerate it. Because this kind of rage is so destructive and so many people are sent to therapy for anger management, the idea of using rage constructively almost never comes up. But rage is one of the antidotes to parasympathetic lockup—where fear conditioning keeps people from realizing their anger, assertiveness, and power. Every coach and drill instructor knows this.

Sandy came to see me for help in "getting his life on track." He was in the process of extricating himself from an emotionally and physically abusive marriage that had gone on for a dozen years. Besides his two young daughters, he could not see anything positive that had come from the relationship, and he felt exhausted and demoralized after so many years of hostile criticism, physical attacks, and what he called emotional sabotage. Beyond laying all of the blame on his soon-to-be ex-wife, he also described a pattern of relating to business associates in the same timid, unassertive, and deferential manner as he had with his wife. Sure that his way of relating had severely damaged his professional success, Sandy realized that there was something within him that severely limited his ability to love and work.

As I got to know Sandy, he described a physically and emotionally abusive father who was a constant source of fear until the time he left home for college. He also described his loyalty to his passive and saintly mother, who tried to hold the family together at the expense of her own physical health and emotional well-being. This led Sandy to identify with his mother and adopt both her religious beliefs and her avoidant behaviors in the face of conflict. He was a deeply conditioned beta, which is why his marriage felt like such a perfect fit for him, much to the horror of his friends and work associates.

The details of his professional life read like a long list of missed opportunities. Sandy was a gifted and creative engineer who had developed a string of inventions with great promise. Each one missed because of his failure to be visible and promote his ideas. He was frightened to approach investors, anxious about making phone calls to important connections, and unable to stand up in front of a group and describe what he had created. "I've avoided anything that might result in conflict or failure," he told me, "which has resulted in conflict and failure."

Sandy told me that whenever he anticipated conflict, he would automatically forget about the situation and move on to something else. "This has resulted in all my accomplishments being negated by the problems I create by avoidance and hiding. Any good will I create gets lost; any money I make ends up paying for the debts I accrue." Sandy's amygdala "believes" that in order for him to survive he has to avoid visibility and anger. Even in the face of all of the pain and failure he has experienced, it has kept him from doing anything different. He has also developed a conscious self-narrative or life story that describes him as a failed beta.

Because the biology of beta status is so primitive, I needed to employ any possible lever to modify the way his brain was wired. His anger, assertiveness, and power had been inhibited, but I wondered whether his primitive rage was still accessible. And if so, was it strong enough to counterbalance his parasympathetic inhibition? How could Sandy activate and harness his primitive rage to help himself break past the fears that held him prisoner? I decided against the machine gun Kelly scenario and tried to think of something closer to his day-to-day experience. Here's what I came up with. I asked Sandy to close his eyes and imagine the following scenario:

LC: On the way home from picking your daughters up at school, you stop for gas. While the car is filling up, the girls ask if they can get a snack, so the three of you walk into the convenience store. As the girls are searching the shelves for snacks, you notice that your seven-year-old, now at the other side of the store, is being grabbed by a man who is trying to pull her out of the store. She calls out, "Daddy, Daddy!"

Before I even ask Sandy what he is thinking and feeling, I can see the tension in his body as he leans forward, and his eyes well up with tears. I ask him what he is experiencing.

S: I'm feeling terrified and enraged at the same time.

LC: What do you feel in your body?

S: I feel my body moving toward my daughter to save her. I can feel the adrenaline pumping through me. I want to tear this guy apart.

LC: What do you imagine you will do when you get to him? Will you ask him nicely to let go of your daughter or let him have her if he refuses your request?

S: Are you kidding! I'm gonna tear his fucking face off like that chimp did to that woman.

LC: What if he is stronger and bigger than you? He may beat you up.

S: There is no way he is taking my daughter as long as I am still breathing. I'll rip the veins out of his neck with my teeth if I have to.

LC: Nice!

This "uncivilized" reaction was alive and well within Sandy. Organized within layers of his primitive brain that may have been even deeper than his shame, it survived untouched by the fear conditioning of his childhood. We all recognize and understand these emotions, and few people would fault him if this situation were real and he did considerable damage to someone trying to abduct his daughter. The laws of the jungle are evoked in these situations and every parent would find him not guilty.

In that moment, it became clear to Sandy that his self-image as a wimp in his personal narrative was not his entire story. I assured him that his primitive alpha energy was alive and well. After all, hadn't I just tapped into it in under 10 seconds with a very basic visualization? He obviously had it on tap whenever he needed it; he just wasn't aware that it sat in his toolbox. To make matters worse, the story he made up about himself told him not even to look for such a thing within him.

I told Sandy, "This is the alpha part of you we need in order to rewire the fear that is stealing your life away from you. You have to care of yourself like you do for your daughter and rip the face off the fear that keeps you trapped in your present life. You have to be absolutely disloyal to your father by being a powerful, good father to yourself, something your own father was incapable of being. You have to be disloyal to your mother by not being a saint—this is war; this is your life you are fighting for."

The truth for all of us is that when we are not allowed to be angry as children, we have to bury our anger. But when we bury our anger, we also bury our assertiveness and our power. This may have been what we needed to survive living with an abusive parent, but it is exactly what we need to change once we escape. In order to change, we have to summon the courage to rage against the machine in our head so we can activate our bodies and emotions. An amygdala can be like an overprotective parent whom you have to break away from in order to have a life.

Beta Beware

A number of costs are associated with changing our social schema. We have to give up some of what may be our most cherished beliefs, such as (1) living in other people's shadows, (2) always having to worry about what others think of us, (3) living in fear of making mistakes, and (4) feeling like frauds. We may even have to sever ties with those who require us to remain betas—friends, spouses, even parents. We may have to work harder, take more risks, and even accept failure when we move out of our safe beta hiding place. It has to be worth it for us to change—but the rewards can be great.

PART THREE

Dissociation and Integration

Applications to Psychotherapy

CHAPTER 11

Anxiety and Stress

Tell your heart that the fear of suffering is worse than the suffering itself.

Paulo Coelho

THE HUMAN BRAIN is an energy hog, using far more of the body's resources than any of our other organs. This big investment is directly tied to our brain's survival value. As organs of adaptation, brains serve animals like us in three basic ways:

1. Brains appraise the social and physical environments for positive and negative value. Is this good to eat? Is that a friendly dog? Should I be walking this close to the edge of the cliff? In other words, the difference between what's good and bad.
2. Brains organize our navigation toward the things we need and away from things we need to avoid. Brains not only organize our abilities to crawl, walk, and swim, they also select the direction, speed, and style in which we move through the world.
3. The results of appraisal and navigation are stored in implicit memory for future use, what our parents called learning from experience. The brain remembers experiences of reward, punishment, and successful strategies in order apply them in the future.

These abilities to appraise, navigate, and learn from experience, and the neural networks that organize them, have coevolved over millions of years. For modern humans, these integrated neural systems function as an integrated whole. When the information embedded within these systems is well matched to our social and physical environments, we are healthy, happy, and able to love and work. People come to psychotherapy when their brains provide them with appraisals, navigational strategies, and learning histories that are poorly matched to their current lives or their aspirations.

Because our brains have become so sophisticated, it is easy to forget that our modern neural systems are deeply interwoven with the primitive survival circuitry dedicated to arousal, stress, and fear. The most primitive subcortical fight-or-flight circuitry, shared with our reptilian ancestors, has been conserved during evolution, and lies at the core of the modern human brain. As the cortex emerged and expanded, these primitive regions evolved to be densely connected with the most highly evolved neural networks. The result is that our sense of safety modulates everything from our ability to attend, concentrate, and learn, to our core beliefs about the world, the future, and ourselves.

Our experiences of anxiety and fear are the conscious emotional appraisals of our brain and body's ongoing detection of threat. At its most adaptive, anxiety encourages us not to step off a curb without looking both ways or to check to see if we signed our tax forms before sealing the envelope. At its least adaptive, anxiety inhibits learning, halts exploration, and keeps us from taking appropriate risks. Anxiety can be triggered by countless conscious and unconscious cues and has the power to shape our behaviors, thoughts, and feelings. Thus, what started out as a simple alarm system has evolved into a nuisance in need of careful management. For those of us who tend to be anxious, our alarm system is like having a smoke detector above a toaster—we get a lot of false alarms.

Just about any kind of stress triggers a range of physiological changes to prepare the body for fight or flight. Energy is mobilized through increased cardiovascular and muscular tone and conserved via the inhibition of digestion, growth, and immune responses. A cascade of biochemical activations occurs in the hypothalamus, pituitary, and adrenal glands as well as higher levels of glucocorticoids, epinephrine, and endogenous opioids. The physiological consequences of stress are particularly relevant to learning because almost every one of them negatively impacts some aspect of attention, concentration, and memory.

As adults, we experience the effects of high levels of sympathetic arousal in situations such as automobile accidents, at crucial moments during sporting events, or during an especially heated debate. This same process may become activated in children and adolescents when they are called upon to speak in class, bullied on the playground, or overwhelmed by conflict at home. Because we are social animals, other people are our primary sources of safety and stress. How others treat us has a direct and continuous impact on our sympathetic arousal.

Psychotherapy is, at its core, a classroom with one student and one teacher. Clients come to therapy to learn more about themselves and how they can develop more adaptive thoughts, feelings, and behaviors. What we are going to explore in the pages ahead is how stress can shut down learning and why a therapist's ability to help a client modulate stress is key to therapeutic success. Because learning depends on plasticity and plasticity is regulated by arousal, the interpersonal regulation of anxiety by the therapist is one of his or her most powerful therapeutic tools. After all, if the brain is turned off to learning, what good is therapy?

The Amygdala, Hippocampus, and Stress

> *The greatest weapon against stress is our ability to choose*
> *one thought over another.*
> William James

As a brief review, the hippocampus is essential for the encoding and storage of conscious learning and memory. It is also extremely sensitive to the negative effects of stress hormones that cause dendritic degeneration, cell death, and inhibited functioning. The amygdala, our central appraisal-processing hub, is our first executive center during both evolution and development, and it plays a central role in emotional learning throughout life. As such, it is a key neural player in associating conscious and unconscious indications of danger with preparation for a survival response. Its central role in environmental appraisal and triggering the biochemical cascade of the fight-or-flight response makes it vital for processing memory, emotional regulation, and attachment.

The neural projections from the amygdala to numerous anatomical targets cause multiple physical expressions of stress, anxiety, and fear. For example, projections from the amygdala to the lateral hypothalamus result in increased heart rate and blood pressure, while those to the trigeminal facial motor nerve trigger fearful facial expressions. One important descending connection from the amygdala projects to the locus coeruleus, the brain's norepinephrine generator. Norepinephrine enhances our focus on danger while inhibiting nonessential activities such as learning new information.

Why is chronic stress so detrimental to our health and well-being? The central mechanism of action is mediated via a group of hormones known as glucocorticoids, specifically cortisol. Glucocorticoids are secreted by the adrenal glands to promote immediate survival. The first aspect of this process that was discovered was the breakdown of complex compounds so that they can be used for immediate energy. The first of these hormones was found to break down complex sugars, hence the name glucocorticoids. This provides for the rapid energy demands of the fight-flight response.

It was later discovered that glucocorticoids play a broader role in the fight-flight response. In addition to their catabolic role in providing instant energy, they also inhibit many of the general maintenance functions of the body. The logic seems to be that if we don't survive the immediate threat, long-term maintenance is a waste of time. Therefore, their other role has been to block protein synthesis or the coming together of simple protein structures involved in the building of the brain and the body.

This doesn't sound detrimental until you take a closer look. When you inhibit protein synthesis, you not only shut down immunological functioning but you also stop the building of new neural structures dedicated to learning. Again, same logic—why protect yourself from infection or learn new information when your life is in danger? This system makes sense for primitive animals that live in simple environments with small imaginations, but not so much for humans.

Neuroscience Corner: The Actions of Cortisol

Breaks down sugars, fats, and proteins for immediate energy

Inhibits neural growth and long-term health

Inhibits inflammatory processes

Inhibits immunological functioning by ceasing production of leukocytes, T cells, natural killer cells, and others

---

The biological link between prolonged stress and hippocampal atrophy appears to be mediated via the catabolic influence of stress hormones. Overall, the mechanisms of long-term well-being are sacrificed for the sake of immediate survival. This strategy makes great sense when stressors are short lived. But when stress is chronic, high levels of cortisol put us at risk of physical illness and deficits of learning and memory.

The human brain is well equipped to survive brief periods of stress without long-term damage. In an optimal state, stressful experiences can be quickly resolved with good coping skills and the help of caring others. Working with rats and vervet monkeys, Robert Sapolsky demonstrated that sustained stress results in hippocampal atrophy and a variety of functional impairments. His research is particularly important because it may help explain some of the negative long-term effects of childhood stress and trauma.

Neuroscience Corner: The Effects of Cortisol on the Hippocampus, Memory, and Learning

Inhibition of neurogenesis, neural growth, and cell maintenance

Degeneration of dendrites, deficits of myelination, and cell death

Impairments in new learning, explicit memory, and spatial reasoning

The consistent high levels of stress and cortisol production generated by the human cortex and modern society are poorly matched to our Paleolithic primitive stress systems. It is apparent that this system was designed to cope with brief periods of stress in emergency situations, not to be maintained for weeks or years at a time. Because of their negative long-term effects, the biological processes related to stress need to be reversed immediately after the crisis has passed in order to allow the body to return to functions of restoration and repair.

Prolonged stress and sustained high levels of glucocorticoids and cortisol disrupts three central processes of the maintenance and building of our brains and bodies. First, by inhibiting protein synthesis in order to maintain higher levels of metabolism, the production of the central building blocks of our immunological systems (e.g., leukocytes, B cells, T cells, natural killer cells) is suppressed. Our diminished capacity to fight off infection and illness is a primary reason for the high correlation between prolonged stress and disease.

Second, because the building of neurons and dendrites also depends upon protein synthesis, sustained levels of stress result in the inhibition of brain growth and impaired learning. Third, sustained stress results in chronically high levels of brain metabolism, which are good in short bursts, but bad if sustained. Continuous stress triggers the pumping of sodium into neurons, which eventually overwhelms the cell's ability to transport it out again. Over time, the neurons become engorged and the cell membrane ruptures, resulting in neuronal death. This process has been found to be particularly damaging to the hippocampus, resulting in a variety of memory deficits and depression. All of these processes disrupt a client's ability to adapt to day-to-day life and to benefit from therapy.

Learning's Sweet Spot

> *The secret of genius is to carry the spirit of the child into old age,*
> *which means never losing your enthusiasm.*
> Aldous Huxley

While we intuitively understand that our clients have to be in a receptive state of mind to engage in psychotherapy, it is actually the state of their brains that allows them to benefit from treatment. The key to a brain that is receptive to learning is the proper balance among hippocampal and amygdala activation, the neural systems they quarterback, and the biological activation they create within the brain. Let's begin with a basic study that relates arousal to learning and work back to psychotherapy from there.

Over a century ago, two researchers named Yerkes and Dodson suspected that a strong relationship existed between learning and arousal. Their hypothesis was that the more you stress animals, the more motivated they will be to learn and hence, the more they will learn. Translated into a research study, the more powerful shock a mouse received as punishment for not learning, the more it would learn. So what they predicted was a one-to-one correspondence between arousal and learning.

Contrary to expectation, they found that mice learned to avoid a moderate shock faster than one of high or low intensity. They charted their findings on a graph with arousal on the x-axis and learning (performance) on the y-axis (see Figure 1). Over the years, the same phenomenon was found to occur in many species, including humans and across an array of learning tasks. Their findings came to be known as the inverted-U learning curve.

The evolutionary logic of this inverted-U relationship between learning and arousal probably goes something like this: When our needs for food, companionship, and safety are satisfied, and nothing interesting is going on, there is no reason

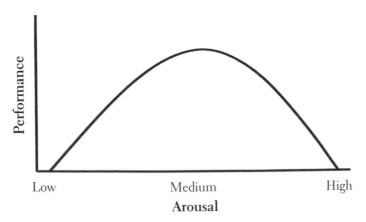

FIGURE 1. The Inverted-U Learning Curve.

to invest energy in learning. Therefore, at low levels of arousal, the amygdala signals the hippocampus to take a break and relax. At the other extreme, dangerous situations call for immediate action and are no time for new cortical learning. At these times, the amygdala also signals the hippocampus and the cortex to stand down so that all available energy can be diverted to bodily survival. These two strategies reflect the left and right sides of the inverted U, respectively.

It is somewhere within these extremes that we find neuroplasticity's sweet spot, that is, where learning is supported through the amygdala's signal to the hippocampus to pay attention and learn. The sweet spot appears to be somewhat to the left of the peak of the curve, a state of arousal we might call motivation, exploration, and curiosity. This state usually contains some risk and a sense of danger, but not enough to trigger a state of defensiveness and withdrawal.

While Yerkes and Dodson's research took place well before we knew much about the neuroscience of learning, this same inverted-U pattern has been found to parallel the underlying biochemistry involved in hippocampal activation. However, this plasticity is inhibited at moderate and high levels of arousal.

At mild levels of arousal, the amygdala enhances hippocampal and cortical plasticity by stimulating the release of moderate levels of norepinephrine and glucocorticoids. Through these chemical messages, the hippocampus is alerted to the importance of remembering what is being experienced and turns on long-term potentiation (LTP), neurogenesis, neural plasticity, and other biological processes involved in learning. Mild amygdala activation facilitates hippocampal and cortical plasticity through protein synthesis, epigenetic transcription, and the activation of neural growth hormones. When we are too anxious or afraid, the amygdala triggers high levels of norepinephrine and cortisol that inhibit hippocampal activation and new learning.

Hippocampal neurons require low levels of cortisol for stimulation and structural maintenance while higher levels of cortisol inhibit their growth and other neuroplastic properties. Cortisol impacts learning and plasticity by regulating the protein synthesis required for dendritic growth and components of neural plasticity, including LTP, long-term synaptic depression (LTD), and primed burst potentiation in this same inverted-U pattern. High levels of stress trigger endorphin release, which impedes both protein synthesis and the consolidation of explicit memory.

Neuroscience Corner: The Bed Nucleus of the Stria Terminalis

A limbic structure closely connected to the amygdala is the bed nucleus of the stria terminalis (BNST). Like the amygdala, it is connected upward to the prefrontal cortex, as well as down into the autonomic nervous system. Unlike the amygdala, the BNST is sensitive to abstract cues and is capable of long-term activation, suggesting both its later evolution and its role in anticipatory anxiety. It appears that the amygdala specializes in fear, while the BNST has evolved to deal with more complex anxiety triggers that emerged as our brains became more capable of future-oriented thinking, such as, "Will I have the money to pay my taxes next April?" The BNST in rats has been found to grow in response to maternal responsibilities. Perhaps this is why many parents mention constant worry as a primary emotion of having children, even before their birth.

As therapists regulate stress levels in the consulting room through their interpersonal and technical skills, they are also manipulating the neuroplastic capabilities of the brains of their clients. We are challenged to keep reminding ourselves that learning is stimulated during times of exploration and adaptation, and turned off by stress and anxiety. We can use these principles to optimize neural plasticity in the service of learning and positive brain change.

Two key correlates of therapeutic success are the quality of the relationship and the reduction in avoidance behavior. A secure relationship both stimulates positive metabolism and regulates anxiety, which assists in keeping the brain in a neuroplastic sweet spot. A reduction in avoidance behavior is an indication that anxiety is being modulated and that the brain has the opportunity to confront what it has associated with a fear response and to learn not to be afraid.

Plasticity in Psychotherapy

> *Things do not change; we change.*
> Henry David Thoreau

An unfortunate twist of evolutionary fate is that the amygdala is mature at birth while the systems that regulate and inhibit it take many years to develop and mature. Thus, we enter the world totally vulnerable to overwhelming fear with no ability to protect ourselves. On the other hand, we are capable of attuning with caretakers who can regulate our fear circuitry until our own brains are ready to take on the job. The way our parents modulate our anxiety and protect us from fear becomes the template upon which our social and emotional neural circuitry becomes organized. This is why we use proximity to our parents during the early years of life as our primary means of emotional regulation. In secure attachment, the child is able to use the parent as a safe haven and avoid experiencing autonomic activation in response to stress. A secure attachment to the therapist allows clients to cope with the stress of new learning and regulate their fear of failure with the therapist's support. It is in this context of safety and autonomic regulation that the brain becomes plastic enough to benefit from most learning situations, especially psychotherapy.

The hippocampus is constantly remodeled to keep up with new learning while the amygdala records and stores threats for future reference. Because the amygdala exhibits persistent dendritic modeling, we are unable to erase the painful or traumatic associations stored within it that lead many of us to be biased toward anxiety and fear. Getting past our fears and phobias appears to require the formation of new descending neural connections from the cortex to the amygdala. These connections are thought to prevent the amygdala from triggering the sympathetic nervous system and the experiences we associate with anxiety, fear, and panic.

Evidence for the power of the cortex to inhibit the amygdala includes their reciprocal activation pattern — more cortical activation results in less amygdala activation and vice versa. The severity of fear and anxiety is also positively associated with amygdala activation and negatively correlated with orbito-medial prefrontal cortex (OMPFC) size and responsivity. It is now believed that it is within the descending networks from the OMPFC to the amygdala's central nucleus that extinction learning is remembered and carries out its inhibitory influences. By experiencing anxiety without harm, our brains learn to change how they respond to feared stimuli. This is the system that is built during successful psychotherapy.

Anxiety and depression are associated with a reduction in top-down control of cues for threat and negative emotions, respectively. These may be some of the reasons why our problem-solving abilities are degraded by fear while preparation for a situation often lessens our fears. And while those of us with more attentional control will still have a bias to orient toward the threat, we will exert more top-down control as we become conscious of the stimulus. Overall, stress, anxiety, and fear are all enemies of learning. They impair cortical processing, problem solving, and the underlying biochemistry of neuroplasticity. Whatever therapists can do to minimize anxiety and stress in themselves and their clients will enhance positive change. Keeping clients in their neuroplastic sweet spot is a core element in therapy.

CHAPTER 12

Understanding and Treating Trauma

How little can be done under the spirit of fear.

Florence Nightingale

STRESS AND TRAUMA are associated phenomena that exist on a spectrum of severity. To understand trauma, you have to first grasp the meaning of stress. But the spectrum of stress and trauma is not traced by a smooth line. Each one of us has a point where anxiety crosses the line to fear and then to terror. When we go from investigating the noise in the other room to seeing someone climbing in the window or moving from fear of blowing an important presentation to having our fear confirmed in the facial expressions of our boss, our minds and bodies mobilize an array of survival responses.

If you feel like a more primitive part of your brain takes over, you would be correct. These ancient responses, conserved from our reptilian ancestors, were designed for far simpler brains for shorter periods of time. As discussed in earlier chapters, one of the great problems created by evolution is embedding this simple system in a very complex brain embedded in a very complex social structure — imagine a five-year-old operating a transit system.

Every biological organism has a set of barriers to regulate the relationship between inner and outer worlds. Our skin defines us as separate from the physical environment while regulating body temperature, keeping out toxic substances, and letting in those things we need to survive. Inside our bodies, our gastrointestinal tract houses vast bacteria colonies that allow us to digest food. Food passes through our intestines, but the bacteria are contained. Surface membranes such as these are formed in different ways throughout our bodies and across the animal kingdom.

In a similar fashion, our psychological, emotional, and social survival depends upon a series of membranes that psychotherapists refer to as defenses and social psychologists call distortions. Like our skin, these defenses and distortions mediate the kind and amount of information allowed into consciousness awareness. They serve survival by regulating anxiety, decreasing the negative impact of failure, and allowing us to create thoughts, feelings, and behaviors that support perseverance in the face of life's more difficult realities. Everyone's defenses, like their immunological systems, vary in strength. Some of us are healthy, robust, and emotionally resilient. Others get sick more often, experience pain and loss too directly, and get knocked down by small slights at every turn.

While some people are resistant to stress and very strong emotionally, it is important to remember that no one is completely immune to trauma. Everyone's defenses have a breaking point, where stress and fear overrun our defenses, and stress turns to terror. This takes us to the notion of the stimulus barrier—the psychological version of the skin. Freud's definition of trauma, as a surpassing of the stimulus barrier, always fascinated me. I understood that he wanted to connect our psychology and biology, but it was hard for me to think of it as more than a metaphor.

By the Way . . .

Don't be surprised that our bodies react to criticism, rejection, and social shaming the same way they do to physical threats—this is because our later-evolving social systems were grafted onto preexisting structures dedicated to physical survival. This is also why pain medications and anti-inflammatories decrease the pain of social rejection—the neural systems of mind, body, self, and others are intertwined.

Trauma: Surpassing the Stimulus Barrier

> *There are very few monsters who warrant the fear we have of them.*
> André Gide

Why are some negative experiences successfully processed and rapidly gotten over while others result in the symptoms of PTSD? What is our stimulus barrier and how is it surpassed? In other words, what are the mechanisms of action of trauma? After many years of working with traumatized clients and studying the brain, answers to these questions slowly began to emerge.

The stimulus barrier can be thought of as a set of homeostatic processes of brain, mind, and relationship that allow us to navigate stress while remaining neurally integrated, conscious of what is happening to us, and connected to those around us. The cortex remains in control; conscious awareness is continuous; and our thoughts, feelings, and behaviors are woven into an ongoing narrative. The stimulus barrier is surpassed when neural systems disconnect from one another, when the continuity of consciousness is replaced with avoidance, denial, and amnesia, and when our ability to remain connected to others becomes fragmented. The cortex becomes inhibited; the integration of our processing systems becomes dissociated, and our narrative fragments.

Neuroscience Corner: The Neurobiological Consequences of Trauma

1. Executive functioning and memory processing are taken over by the amygdala.
2. Cortical executive functions of the frontal and parietal lobes are actively inhibited.
3. The neurobiology of the fight-flight response drives the body, mind, and emotions.
4. Left frontal regions that control language and narrative are inhibited.
5. Social brain systems are disrupted and/or inhibited.
6. Information processing is biased toward the past and the detection of threat.
7. Chronic threat disrupts sympathetic-parasympathetic balance.

Overall, it means that our ability to navigate our physical and social environments in a flexible and coherent manner has been undermined. This is the result of a dissociation of our neurobiological functioning secondary to the effects of overwhelming stress. That is, we—and our brains—flip out. The inhibition of the cortical regions that coordinate conscious awareness leaves the traumatized individual drowning in a sea of fragmented and overwhelming emotions, sensations, and frightening thoughts.

By the Way . . .

The *DSM*'s attempt to define trauma is helpful but far from complete. The complexities of human experience are missed by the reduction to categories and definitions sought by the APA, the AMA, and the pharmaceutical companies. Therefore, go beyond the definitions to the life experiences of your clients to assess whether or not they have experienced trauma and are suffering from the effects.

Posttraumatic Stress Disorder

To him who is in fear, everything rustles.
Sophocles

Trauma can result in a range of interpersonal, physiological, and psychological reactions that have been observed throughout recorded history. Combat experiences, the loss of a child, and natural disasters have been paired with changes in behavior, personality, and relationships throughout the world's literature. Trauma causes a predictable set of symptoms to emerge that tend to gradually diminish after the resolution of the threatening situation. This process of natural healing is a combination of the passage of time, social support, physiological reregulation, and the reestablishment of healthy psychological defenses.

Sometimes, prolonged anxiety, fear, and terror cause severe disturbances in the integration of cognitive, sensory, and emotional processing. As a general rule, the earlier, more severe, and more prolonged the trauma, the more negative and far reaching its effects. Sustained unresolved trauma may result in symptoms of posttraumatic stress disorder (PTSD). PTSD has four groups of symptoms: social fragmentation, hyperarousal, intrusion, and avoidance, reflecting the seven physiological processes described above.

Social fragmentation results from a disruption of attunement, resonance, and empathy secondary to the inhibition of neural systems dedicated to social connection and self-awareness. Symptoms of social fragmentation include difficulties with intimacy, emotional regulation in close relationships, and disruptions of personal identity. This results in clients being unable to benefit from the curative factors gained in personal relationships and makes the establishment of a therapeutic relationship more difficult.

Hyperarousal reflects a stress-induced hyperactivation of the amygdala and autonomic nervous system, resulting in an exaggerated startle reflex, agitation, anxiety, and irritability. That jumpy feeling we get when we drink too much caffeine gives us a taste of this experience. One of the key elements in treatment is to include strategies and techniques to decrease arousal through activities such as biofeedback and relaxation techniques.

Intrusions occur when implicit traumatic memories break into conscious awareness and are experienced as if they are happening in the present. Intrusions may also manifest in nightmares or flashbacks. A combat veteran may hit the deck when a car backfires, or a rape victim may have a panic attack while making love to her husband because she is triggered by a sensory or emotional cue. Psychoeducation about memory system storage can be important in providing a cognitive framework for understanding these "irrational reactions."

Avoidance is the attempt to defend against dangers by limiting contact with the world, withdrawing from others, and narrowing the range of thoughts and feelings. Avoidance can also take the form of denial, repression, dissociation, and amnesia. A focus of therapy is always to make approaching the feared stimulus a priority after the development of new skills to manage physiological fear and arousal.

When experienced in combination, these four groups of symptoms result in a cycle of activation and numbing, reflecting the body's memory for, and continued victimization by, the trauma. Instead of serving to mobilize the body to deal with new external threats, traumatic memories continually trigger frightening emotional responses. An inability to engage in intimate relationships cuts off the primary mechanism of healing trauma and traps the victim in an isolated and frightening inner world.

The Neurochemistry of PTSD

> *It is not death that a man should fear, but he should fear*
> *never beginning to live.*
> Marcus Aurelius

Acute stress and trauma result in predictable patterns of biochemical changes that are part of the body's mobilization to confront threat. Because of this, it is important both to be aware of and to teach our clients what happens in our bodies when we feel threatened. Most people don't realize that these biochemical changes have such a profound effect on their experiences. This lack of knowledge makes victims more vulnerable to attributing their symptoms to character flaws or supernatural causes. This knowledge will positively impact your client's ability to engage in and benefit from therapy.

While knowing the exact biochemistry is not important, having any explanatory model for what we are experiencing activates cortical processes that help to inhibit the amygdala. Having and giving your clients a rationale for what is happening in their brains and minds is a key component of being an amygdala whisperer.

Fear triggers increases in certain biochemical and neurohormones in order to pump up our energy, heighten our vigilance, and make us less susceptible to pain. This system, a holdover from our primitive relatives, is designed for rapid activation to deal with a life-threatening situation that will pass in a minute or two. When stress and trauma are prolonged or become chronic, these neurochemical changes result in long-term alterations that impact all aspects of life. Each of the five neurochemicals has its own role in the stress response and contributes in different ways to the long-term effects of PTSD.

Neuroscience Corner:
The Neurochemistry of PTSD

The increased levels of norepinephrine seen in PTSD prepare us for fight-or-flight readiness and reinforce the biological encoding of traumatic memory. Higher long-term levels of norepinephrine result in an increase in arousal, anxiety, irritability, and a heightened or unmodulated startle response. Besides being stronger, the startle response is also more resistant to habituation in response to subsequent milder and novel stressors. Being consistently startled increases the victim's experience of the world as an unsettling and dangerous place, a good example of a feedback loop between physiological and psychological processes.

Low levels of serotonin found in PTSD correlate with irritability, anxiety, aggression, and depression. Serotonin is a neurotransmitter related to a sense of connection to others, safety, and well-being. Lower levels are associated with separation, hunger, and danger.

Lower levels of serotonin have been found in traumatized humans and animals after they are subjected to inescapable shock. Chronically low levels of serotonin are correlated with higher levels of irritability, depression, suicidality, arousal, and violence.

High levels of dopamine, which can occur in PTSD, correlate with hypervigilance, paranoia, and perceptual distortions in those under stress. Symptoms of social withdrawal and the avoidance of new and unfamiliar situations (neophobia) are shaped by these biochemical changes.

Elevated levels of endogenous opioids, which serve as analgesics to relieve pain in fight-or-flight situations, can have a profoundly negative impact on cognitive function, memory, and reality testing. Higher opioid levels can result in emotional blunting, dissociation, depersonalization, and derealization, all of which provide a sense of distance from the traumatized body. However, these processes become harmful when used as defenses, disrupting our ability to stay engaged in our day-to-day lives.

Sustained high levels of glucocorticoids have a catabolic effect on the nervous system and are thought to be responsible for memory deficits related to decreased hippocampal volume. Glucocorticoids sacrifice long-term conservation and homeostasis for short-term survival. Chronically high levels have negative effects on brain structures and the immune system, resulting in higher rates of learning disabilities and physical illness, which enhances victims' experience of being fragile and vulnerable individuals.

These biochemical changes are paralleled by such symptomatology as emotional dyscontrol, social withdrawal, and lower levels of adaptive functioning. Together, these and other negative effects of trauma result in compromised functioning in many areas of life. The impact of trauma depends on a complex interaction of the physical and psychological stages of development during which it occurs, the length and degree of the trauma, and the presence of vulnerabilities or past traumas. The impact of chronic trauma becomes woven into the structure of personality and is hidden behind other symptoms, making it difficult to identify, diagnose, and treat. One of the underlying mechanisms of action of successful psychotherapy with victims of stress and trauma is to alter these biochemical processes. Any way you can find to decrease arousal will result in lowering the levels of all five of these neurochemicals. Consider using biofeedback and relaxation tapes as part of your treatment plan and supporting activities that serve the same purpose—yoga, playing music, or whatever works for a particular client.

Remembering and Neural Reintegration

Fear is static that keeps me from hearing myself.
Samuel Butler

Memory and consciousness are so interwoven that many feel that consciousness is an evolutionary by-product of the expansion of our working memory. That is, what we label consciousness is the updating of moment-to-moment memory interspersed with memories from the past. This would solve the problem of coming up with a good definition of consciousness separate from what we already understand. And who knows, consciousness may simply be an outgrowth of multiple interwoven memory systems that creates the illusion of an observer. That's too big of a question for me to tackle.

What we do know is that we have multiple memory systems, both conscious and unconscious, that combine in a more or less integrated way to support appraisal, navigation, and learning. We also know that when we are terrified, and arousal gets too high, there is a dissociation of conscious and unconscious systems of memory (an oversimplification that will do for now). This split has been known about since the early days of hypnosis, Freud's residency under Charcot in Paris before he created psychoanalysis, and studied in depth by experimental psychologists for many decades.

The question for psychotherapists has always been how to reconnect dissociated memory systems. Early theories of regression, and later primal screaming, have given way to more measured interventions focused on a balanced dose of uncovering, processing, and support. Freud's goal of expanding conscious awareness has continued to be the coin of the realm, with many ways of getting to the castle.

An interesting strategy for accessing and integrating memory systems is a type of therapy called Eye Movement Desensitization and Reprogramming (EMDR). Like many other forms of treatment, EMDR consists of exposing the client to feared memories in a structured, sensitive, and caring manner. But unlike other methods, it adds a series of eye movements or other forms of sensory stimulation to the process. I dismissed it for a long time because it seemed somewhat faddish, and I thought that waving a finger in a client's face seemed unbecoming for a professional. There was also a certain strange and cultlike feel to the whole thing that put me off. In my decades of doing therapy, I had seen hundreds of fads come and go, and I was waiting for this one to go away as well. Not only did it not go away, but clinicians I respected began saying positive things about it.

As I sidled up to considering EMDR as a legitimate treatment modality, I learned that, other than the eye movements, it appeared to be a basic exposure paradigm, something similar to what I had been taught in systematic desensitization.

So I went into EMDR with a basic question—do the eye movements, finger tapping, or other sensory signals add anything to existing exposure methods? I share my thoughts and experiences here not to promote EMDR or to turn the focus of the book to a how-to manual, but because I believe that my experience of EMDR adds insight into how any therapy works.

The Orienting Reflex and the Reconsolidation of Memory

> *The mark of fear is not easily removed.*
>
> Ernest Gaines

Plenty of research points to the fact that the way information and memory is processed in the brains of those suffering with PTSD is disrupted. We know that our clients tend to narrow their range of behaviors, activities, and emotions out of fear of being unexpectedly triggered by running into something novel, a symptom called neophobia.

When nontraumatized people experience something new, an area of the brain called the anterior cingulate puts them on alert to pay attention and to be prepared to react to and learn from something unexpected. It could be good or bad—we don't know—but if we are not afraid, the curiosity and exploratory urge counterbalance the fear of the unknown. For those with PTSD, the circuits that prepare them for novelty and new learning are not activated. Regions of the brain that organize autobiographical and somatic memory fire instead. Thus, neophobia is actually a fear of being reminded of the pain and terror of the past. In other words, the brains of PTSD victims become shut off from both new learning and the ability to update past experiences.

Our memory and motor systems have been engaged in collaborative evolutionary processes since we were fish. One piece of evidence for this is that when we use the large muscles of our legs to walk or run, they secrete neural growth factors that cross the blood-brain barrier and stimulate neuroplasticity and learning. This connection is most likely due to the fact that our muscles evolved to tell our brains to pay attention when we are moving because something important is happening—otherwise, why would we be moving?

In a similar fashion, side-to-side eye movements likely trigger systems for memory updating because they are historically related to foraging and looking out for predators and prey. This is probably why rapid eye movement (REM) sleep occurs while our brains are engaging in the consolidation of new memory. We don't need to move our eyes to consolidate memory; it is just an artifact of the coevolution of foraging, the orienting response, eye movements, and needing to update our map of our territory.

Neuroscience Corner: Orienting Reflex

The orienting reflex is our automatic response to shift our focus to something that catches our attention. This primitive reflex is seen in all animals as an adaptive response to their environments. As memory systems evolved, it is likely that they were networked with the orienting reflex to signal the brain to get ready to learn new information. This may be the key to the impact of eye movements and other sensory stimulation in EMDR.

Because side-to-side eye movements are evolutionarily significant in their own right, it is likely then that EMDR can activate the orienting reflex through multiple sensory modalities. It is also likely that the orienting reflex counteracts the tendency in the brains of people with PTSD to go back to autobiographical memory in the face of new information. Stimulating the orienting reflex through eye movements or tapping the legs activates the brain's novelty detection centers and allows for memory reconsolidation. This allows new information in and old information to be updated and modified. When EMDR works, I suspect this may be the mechanism of action. You might say that EMDR is a way to trick the brains of individuals with PTSD to process new experiences in a manner that allows them to live in the present.

An important addition here is that I don't think you have to have PTSD to benefit from EMDR. I say that because I think that all of us have had terrifying experiences that we have suppressed, but they still interfere with optimal functioning in certain areas of our lives. This isn't a vague theory, but is based on some personal experience.

Taking the EMDR Plunge

> *A person's fears are lighter when the danger is at hand.*
> Seneca

A couple of years ago, Francine Shapiro, the founder of EMDR, kindly invited me to join an EMDR training to learn more of what it was all about. I sat through the lectures, which were very much in line with what I had read in her books. It all seemed like fairly standard knowledge and accepted Cognitive-Behavioral Therapy, with the addition of sensory stimulation.

No theory was presented for why the eye movements aided treatment, just that they appeared to have clinical utility. This was okay with me—plenty of treatments have been used for centuries without understanding why they work. By the end of the lectures, I was still skeptical of whether the eye movements added anything to the basic exposure therapy that framed them.

Our general instructions were to introduce a problematic situation and interweave sets of 24 to 36 eye movements with gentle encouragement along the way and to use words that imply a somewhat passive stance toward what the client is experiencing, as if watching a movie. Phrases like "just notice that," or "just think of that" were used as expressions of gentle guidance and encouragement. The overall assumption seemed to be that cleaning out the negative would allow for the emergence of the positive. As you stop living your trauma, you begin to live your life.

Before the sessions began, we were instructed to think of time and awareness as scenes viewed from a train and to learn to watch what goes by us. The eye movements signal the brain to focus on the present, and we were cautioned to avoid engaging in talk therapy. Instead of making interpretations based on psychodynamic processes, the EMDR therapist is told to trust the healing process of the brain and mind.

After lunch we divided into groups of four to practice the EMDR treatment that we had learned during the morning lecture. Our job was to go though the protocol with one another in a round robin fashion to get some initial practice. The protocol consisted of going through the steps of asking questions, identifying targets to focus on, and leading our "clients" through the eye movements. As dyad clients, we were to come up with some troubling thing in our life that we wanted to work on. Untypically for me, I couldn't immediately come up with a half dozen things that were bothering me. I was a bit surprised because I've always felt in constant turmoil. I reflected that perhaps all the years of therapy had begun to pay off. Wanting to be of service to my partner, I strained to come up with something that she could work with. If nothing else, I am driven to be a good boy. As I scanned my mind, I realized that I had a monthly faculty meeting coming up and immediately had a negative emotional reaction at the thought of it. I almost always find these meetings boring and annoying, often difficult to tolerate, and sometimes downright painful. I figured that this was something immediate that I could work with that had some emotion attached to it that might yield something, if not important for me, at least a good exercise for my partner.

My first step was to become aware of some of the thoughts and feelings that were associated with the faculty meetings just beneath the surface of the ones I already described. So I imagined sitting in the meetings and reflecting on my experiences of them. I immediately became agitated, annoyed, and wanted to flee. Why do the meetings bother me so much? After all, it is part of my job. They are just a couple of hours a month, and I like everyone in the meetings. For decades, I have been annoyed with the fact that they are poorly run and accomplish very little. By bringing lots of work to do, I can accomplish the same work I could do in my office. Objectively, there was no good reason for me to have such a negative reaction to these meetings. Yet my anxiety, agitation, and impulse to flee were undeniable. Here is my experience of EMDR.

1. As I allowed myself to sink into the feelings I have at the meetings and saw what came up, I began to feel more and more anxious. As I thought about why, what came to my mind was that no one wanted me there. They thought that I was an annoying, self-centered fool who wanted all of the attention. As I continued the exercise, I noticed other thoughts coming to the surface like, "They wish I wasn't there," "They don't take anything I say seriously," "They think of me as an annoying child."

Eye Movements

2. As I thought about my experience in these meetings more objectively, I realized that my negative emotions may have contributed to behaviors that helped turn some of these fears into realities. To cope with my anxiety, I have to distract myself by bringing work or by employing the same defenses I used as a kid to take care of myself—humor, hyperactivity, withdrawal, and avoidance.

Eye Movements

3. As I describe and imagine being in the faculty meeting, I get more in touch with my bodily sensations and emotions. As I allow myself to get deeper into these feelings, I notice that the scene in my mind spontaneously shifts to another from my childhood. Although the context and the characters were different, the feelings mapped perfectly onto the faculty meeting. Now, I have the same feeling in my body and exactly the same emotions, but I am no lon-

ger actively invoking a scene. I am watching this movie playing in my head. I'm in the living room of my grandparents' house sometime in the 1950s. I'm sitting on a sofa across from my mother, grandmother, and grandfather as they look at me attentively. Their faces reflect enthusiasm, interest, and love, and they appear very interested in what I have to say. I am somehow aware that I am soothing the deep pain that they share. My post hoc analysis: I am the magical child who arrived to save them from their depression and despair—the making of a compulsive caretaker. My connection with them feels blissful. I feel that I am bringing them joy.

Eye Movements

4. When the third set of eye movements is complete, I eagerly go back to that special feeling of having all eyes on me. This time there is the addition of a noise in the distance and the sound of footsteps entering the house. It is my father, in his mid-20s, all testosterone, irritability, and anger. His head and face are much larger than those of the other three, and his expression is half angry lion and half hungry hyena. He stalks behind my mother and grandparents, keeping his eyes on me. I am terrified; I know that he hates me and wants me dead—he wants to eat me. When they turn to look at him, he smiles at me. When they turn back to me, his expression once again becomes threatening. My therapist and I are surprised at the emotional power of this image, but it is certainly in line with the his-

tory of our relationship. He encouraged me to enlist in the army during the Vietnam War.

Eye Movements

5. Back at my grandparents' house, I'm sitting across from my mother and grandparents and watch my father stalking behind them. I feel hesitant to get back into the frightening emotions and try to think about it more objectively. As I watch him walk back and forth, I think about how little attention his parents and wife show him relative to how much attention they show me. I think that he is still a young man who needs his father, who was always very tough on him—but who gives me all of his attention. As I thought these thoughts within the scene, I felt as if both my child self and my adult self were sitting together. In fact, the therapist in me was explaining what was happening and, without having to say it, was telling me that my father's hatred of me wasn't about me at all.

It was at this point that I began to experience a difference in this form of treatment. My experience of session five was less like doing the work of therapy and more like witnessing the therapy happening. It was akin to my experience of writing, where once a character has been developed in my mind, I shift from having to think about what he should do next to transcribing what I see him doing in my mind's eye—a process that is reflected with the gentle prompting of "just notice that" or "just think of that" that EMDR folks use during sessions.

Eye Movements

6. Going back again to the scene, I noticed that this time my father's head was smaller and that his face was now his own. His expression was no longer menacing but sad, crestfallen, and despairing. I also noticed that I no longer felt as good about being the recipient of all of this attention at his expense. In fact, it almost seemed that the attention I was getting was a way of punishing him. I had aged quickly in this scenario. I was no longer the child soaking up attention, but was embarrassed about willingly playing along with this destructive family scenario. I had been trapped in this family drama, and we had all paid the price. Somewhere near the end of this sequence, I turned to my grandfather, pointed to my father, and said, "Your son needs you."

Two things about this experience were quite compelling. The first was that instead of working hard to rethink and reorganize my memory, it was if I was watching these internal events taking place on a screen. The six stages of experience I describe unfolded before me as if I was a witness as opposed to the central character, very much like a dream state. The second compelling aspect of the experience was that in the faculty meeting in the week that followed, I felt unburdened of the extreme emotions that had plagued me in the past. The meeting was as boring and nonproductive as ever, but clear of the baggage that I always brought in with me. I was impressed with the results—EMDR had opened a new window in the world of memory.

While we tend to think of memory as a well-organized filing cabinet or digital files on a hard drive, the reality is much more complex, reflecting a long and convoluted history of the brain, body, mind, and social relatedness. A more accurate image for a human memory would be that each memory consists of a puzzle with its pieces stored across the country based on some complex, nonlinear formula that we have yet to decode. We also possess multiple systems of memory that can either be integrated or dissociated. As a result of trauma, memory systems can fragment from each other, resulting in dissociation.

Trauma: The Gift That Keeps on Giving

Men are not prisoners of fate, but only prisoners of their own minds.
Franklin D. Roosevelt

We have all heard the sayings "What doesn't kill you makes you stronger" and "Time heals all wounds." These bits of common wisdom conjure up pictures of difficult and traumatic experiences that, once overcome, result in greater levels of physical and emotional well-being. Although trials and tribulations can certainly be important learning experiences, they can also create long-standing biological and psychological compromise. Trauma can produce chronic biological, psychological, and social damage that can interfere with all levels of functioning. So in the case of chronic and severe trauma, "What doesn't kill you can make you weaker." Just ask the relatives of combat veterans, Holocaust survivors, or victims of childhood sexual abuse.

Unfortunately, trauma is a gift that keeps on giving. The more trauma you have experienced, the more likely it is that you will be traumatized again. And the more trauma you have experienced, the more likely you are to develop PTSD after a subsequent trauma. Increased stress secondary to trauma also decreases immunological functioning, making it more likely that traumatized individuals will suffer from physical illnesses. All of these findings are especially true if you experienced trauma early in life over a sustained period of time. Understanding and healing trauma is an important focus of our work, one that we need to continue expanding and deepening.

CHAPTER 13

Complex Trauma: A Developmental Perspective

The other day I heard someone knocking on my window.
I'd rather be dead than hear that.
A 10-year-old kidnapping victim

FOR THE GENERAL public, the idea of trauma is interwoven with images from the 11 o'clock news: accidents, assaults, combat, terrorism, and natural disasters—the money shot of every news broadcast. The field of mental health long held the same focus. From the victims of industrial accidents of nineteenth-century Europe through the thousands of shell-shocked veterans from the world wars, our thinking about trauma has been shaped by the effects of traumatic experiences on well-functioning adults. For obvious reasons, we find it harder to think of children being traumatized—especially at the hands of those who are supposed to love and protect them.

Although we like to think of childhood as a time of innocence and safety, many children grow up with stress and trauma. Into the 1990s, surgery was performed on infants without anesthesia, and still less than 25% of physicians performing circumcision on newborns use any form of analgesia. These practices appear to be a holdover of beliefs that newborns either don't experience or don't remember pain. Parental physical or mental illness, community violence, poverty, and many other factors can also be sources of sustained stress and trauma. For a young child, separation from parents, looking into the eyes of a depressed mother, or living in a highly stressful household can also be traumatic. For an African American adolescent, institutionalized prejudice and hopelessness about a better future could also qualify. And what about an elderly widower who loses the dog that he and his wife adopted together many years ago? Bottom line, there are no objective criteria for what constitutes stress or trauma. The existence of trauma has to be assessed on a case-by-case basis with an open mind and an open heart.

Very Early Stress

> *Fate chooses our relatives, we choose our friends.*
> Jacques Delille

As an organ of adaptation, during gestation the brain begins to be shaped to the world it is preparing to enter. While brain stem development relies on the programming within our DNA, limbic and cortical development depend largely on the influence of experience on genetic expression. That is, experience builds our brains to optimize adaptation and survival to whatever environment our mothers signal to us we are about to enter.

One example of this is how a mother's stress shapes the brain of her unborn child via their shared biochemistry. Maternal stress tells the fetal brain that the world is a dangerous place. Although this helps prepare the baby for a dangerous world, it also makes him or her more susceptible to anxiety, immune suppression, and learning difficulties for all of the reasons discussed in the last two chapters. A sad example of this intergenerational transfer is the fact that children of traumatized parents have an increased prevalence of PTSD, most likely because they were primed from the beginning to experience the world as a dangerous and untrustworthy place.

Another example is maternal depression, which serves as a highly stressful challenge for infants and children. After all, infants depend on their mothers for survival, and a deflated, slowed, and emotionless mother is a huge risk to survival. Depressed mothers are angry with and disengage from their infants more often, are more likely to physically poke them, and spend less time in matching emotional states. Although we would not consider these infants traumatized in the traditional sense, the loss of maternal resonance, engagement, and vitality are all experienced as life threatening by a totally dependent infant.

It is not surprising that infants of depressed mothers show many signs of depression themselves, including increased right frontal cortical activation and higher norepinephrine levels, heart rates, and cortisol levels. Just like their depressed mothers, these infants engage in fewer interactive behaviors that are vital for their healthy neural and social development.

Complex Posttraumatic Stress Disorder

> *A child understands fear and the hurt and hate it brings.*
> Nadine Gordimer

The effects of early and severe trauma are extremely widespread, devastating, and difficult to treat. Because of the importance of a context of safety and bonding in the early construction of the brain, childhood trauma compromises the healthy development of core neural networks. It stands to reason that the most devastating types of trauma are those that occur at the hands of caretakers. Physical and sexual abuse by parents not only traumatizes children, but also deprives them of healing interactions and of having a safe haven. The wide range of effects involved in the adaptation to early unresolved trauma results in complex PTSD.

Definition: Complex PTSD

Complex PTSD occurs in the context of early, prolonged, and inescapable trauma, often at the hands of parents or caretakers. It is called complex because of its effects on a child's physiological, psychological, and social development. The enduring personality traits and coping strategies that emerge in these situations tend to decrease positive adaptation and increase an individual's vulnerability to future trauma. This can manifest through engagement in abusive relationships, poor judgment, or a lack of adequate self-protection.

In essence, the personality and character of children with complex PTSD develop in the shadow of trauma, and they never appear to make the developmental and evolutionary leap from amygdala to cortical executive functioning. Their lives are lived in a survival-based, amygdala-centric manner, and they are less connected to the consensual realities of the group mind. They are, in essence, a more primitive version of modern humans—yet are tasked to live among others whose brains are organized in a fundamentally different way.

For an adult under normal circumstances, a threat triggers a fight-or-flight response. The threat is dealt with, and the flight-fight response soon subsides. Children are not well equipped to cope with threat in this way. Fighting and fleeing may actually be maladaptive because their survival depends on relying on those around them. When a child experiences trauma inflicted by a caretaker, or cries for help but no help arrives, he or she may shift from fear and hyperarousal to psychological and neurological numbing and dissociation. Children depend on a safe connection with adults to help them learn to regulate their anxiety, shifting from amygdala to cortical control.

Don't simply check off the boxes in an intake report indicating "all developmental milestones reported to have been met on time"; find out about the environments in which clients developed—a mother's postpartum depression, a grandmother's violent death, a father's unemployment. Factors like these, critical to psychological development, if missed, can lead to years of confusion in therapy. With secure attachment, the child is able to use the parent as a safe haven and to avoid experiencing autonomic activation in response to stress. A secure attachment in the therapeutic relationship allows a client to confront challenges in therapy, making it a "safe emergency" in which to learn and grow.

Dissociation allows the traumatized individual to escape the trauma via a number of biological and psychological processes. Derealization and depersonalization reactions allow the victim to avoid the reality of his or her situation, or watch it as a detached observer. Hyperarousal and dissociation in childhood create an inner biopsychosocial environment primed to establish boundaries between different emotional states and experiences. Compulsive disorders related to eating or gambling, somatization disorders in which emotions are converted into physical symptoms, and borderline personality disorder (BPD) all reflect varieties of complex adaptations to early trauma.

Borderline Personality Disorder as Early Attachment Trauma

> *All my life, my heart has yearned for a thing I cannot name.*
> André Breton

It is popular to argue about the legitimacy and usefulness of the BPD diagnosis. Does it reflect a true pathological process or a culturally embedded prejudice against women? Regardless of the underlying reality, the symptoms associated with the diagnosis of BPD are extremely interesting from the perspective of early attachment and brain development. Adults diagnosed with BPD do report higher levels of childhood trauma, physical and emotional abuse, and lower levels of parental care than those with other psychiatric diagnoses.

A number of clinicians have made the case that what we call BPD is one developmental outcome of early, persistent, and unresolved trauma. Dr. Bessel van der Kolk has made a compelling argument for the idea that BPD, somatization disorder, dissociative identity disorders, and alexithymia are different expressions of early traumatic experiences. Clients with these diagnoses tend to share difficult histories and suffer from anxiety, identity disturbances, blocked affect, and severe emotional and cognitive dysregulation similar to that seen in PTSD.

The degree of symptom severity in adulthood appears to correlate with the severity and chronicity of stress, abuse, and trauma during childhood. Dissociators employ the imaginative capacities of the frontal lobes to shut off the experience of emotional pain, creating alternate experiences, worlds, and identities. Those with PTSD suffer from the oscillating dysregulation of emotional arousal when cued by either conscious or unconscious associations.

During memories of childhood trauma, adult women with BPD have been shown to fail to activate prefrontal and anterior cingulate regions, like those with PTSD. Somatizers and alexithymics demonstrate a disconnection between the cognitive and emotional processing centered in the left and right cortices. Alexithymia in adulthood correlates with being an unwanted child, and attachment patterns tend to be insecure, either avoidant-dismissing or preoccupied and fearful.

Attachment trauma can result from physical or sexual abuse, neglect, or profound misattunement between parent and child. Affective disorders have also been shown to occur at above-average rates in these patients and their parents, a likely contributing factor to difficulties in emotional regulation. Whatever the cause, the child is unable to utilize others in the development of secure attachment and to regulate overwhelming anxiety and fear. The result is that real or imagined abandonment triggers a state of terror, similar to what any young primate experiences when physically abandoned by its mother.

What we witness in the lives of clients with BPD appears to be the result of the disruption of the development and integration of social brain and other neural systems that impair emotional regulation, interpersonal experience, and executive functioning. It is most likely that the symptoms of BPD are the outcome of an interaction between their innate neurobiology and the effects of life experiences on their brain, mind, and spirit. Examining the process of the brain's adaptation to early interpersonal trauma may provide a way of understanding BPD that will help to better treat this painful and debilitating social disorder.

The Borderline Brain

> *Life without love is like a tree without blossoms.*
> Khalil Gibran

There is considerable evidence of abnormal neural development in the brains of clients with BPD that impacts their cognitive, emotional, and interpersonal functioning. These clients show abnormalities in size, activation patterns, and neurochemical levels in several brain regions including the hippocampus, amygdala, and left orbital medial and right anterior cingulate cortices. As we might expect, the ways in which borderline brains differ from brains of nonpatients are found in networks of the social brain and those involved in regulating impulses, emotions, and social relationships.

Neuroscience Corner: Patients With BPD Exhibit Volume Reduction

Brain Region	Related Function
Frontal and prefrontal lobes	Executive functioning and affect regulation
Amygdala	Affect recognition and abandonment anxiety
Hippocampus	Reality testing and short-term memory consolidation
Anterior cingulate cortex	Integration of cognitive and emotional processing
Posterior cingulate cortex	Sensory processing
Parietal cortex (right)	Executive processing and somatic awareness
Corpus callosum (women)	Integration of cognition and emotion

At rest, the brains of borderline patients demonstrate hypometabolism in prefrontal and anterior cingulate cortices and show hypoarousal on measures of heart rate, skin conductance, and pain sensitivity. But when the same subjects are shown slides of emotionally adverse situations, they show greater activation in the amygdala, the prefrontal, temporal, and occipital cortex, and the fusiform gyrus. Simultaneously, the hippocampus, which is required for reality testing, new learning, and amygdala modulation, becomes less active.

Of special note are deficits of visual processing and visual memory, given the strong ties between the amygdala and the visual cortex. This may be why there is such a high comorbidity of BPD and body dysmorphic disorder. Amygdala activation and its connections to primary visual areas may distort the fundamental perception of faces and bodies, both our own and others'. These clients demonstrate higher amygdala and visual processing network activation in processing negative emotional stimuli than normal. In other words, they activate more primitive networks when confronted with negative stimuli. The trauma resulting from interpersonal betrayal appears to be particularly salient in their minds, and they tend to see the world as more malevolent and themselves as sufferers of bad fortune.

Traditional neuropsychological testing demonstrates deficits in executive function, attention, memory, and a variety of cognitive processes, similar to neurology patients with frontal and temporal lobe damage. This is important to remember because treatment has to be modified to account for these cognitive limitations. Like other clients with PTSD, intrusive emotions lead them to operate many IQ points below capacity. Although they may be very intelligent when unstressed, their cognitive abilities decrease when stressed. The result is repeated treatment failures, negative transference reactions, and ruptures of attunement. One of the key reasons why dialectical behavior therapy is successful is because it scaffolds clients in a way that compensates for deficits in cognitive and emotional processing, which is central to the disorder.

The Social Brain of the Borderline

> *Sometimes I feel my whole life has been one big rejection.*
> Marilyn Monroe

Research has found that clients with BPD tend to read happy faces accurately but misinterpret or exaggerate neutral and negative ones. They are more likely to see disgust and surprise and miss expressions of fear in the faces of others. Thus, there is a tendency to both negatively distort neutral information and take it personally, a primary reason why these errors in reading facial expression correlate with antagonism, suspiciousness, and assaultiveness. This may be why we see these individuals having so many deficits in social problem solving when neutral or negative emotions are involved.

Clients with BPD are highly sensitive to rejection of any kind, evidenced in a higher level of amygdala activation in general. They also show higher anterior cingulate activation when witnessing pictures of people facing stressful situations alone or being socially excluded. Memories of abandonment are associated with increased bilateral activation in the dorsolateral prefrontal cortex and decreases in right anterior cingulate activation.

The bottomless well of need in borderline individuals may in part be due to a deficit in the ability to feel taken care of at a primitive, visceral level. Such a deficit could be due to inborn genetic variables such as deficits of serotonin or oxytocin activation or experience-dependent shaping of basal forebrain circuits during early attachment relationships. These findings suggest that their brains are on high alert for danger, and misjudge and distort incoming information, while simultaneously decreasing inhibition, reality testing, and emotional control. All of these parallel the struggles of clients with traditional PTSD.

When clients with BPD experience negative feelings, they are overwhelmed and unable to use the conscious cortical processing needed to test the appropriateness of their reactions or to solve whatever problems they are facing. They lose perspective, the ability to remember ever feeling good, or the idea that they may ever feel good again. Overwhelming fear and lack of perspective combine to create the experience that their very life is at risk.

Clients with BPD demonstrated low serotonin synthesis and diminished serotonin regulation in their prefrontal, temporal, and parietal cortices. These findings correlate with the increased impulsivity, depression, difficulty being soothed, and decreased emotional inhibition seen in these patients. They also have heightened or unstable levels of norepinephrine, triggered by unregulated activation of the amygdala. A number of neurotransmitter systems within the social brain, including serotonin, norepinephrine, dopamine, and GABA, as well as abnormalities of vagal regulation, are most likely involved in affective and behavioral instability.

Like those suffering with PTSD, clients with BPD are often anxious, hyperaroused, and vulnerable to depression. Adolescents with BDP and PTSD have been found to have smaller pituitary glands, which may reflect chronic dysregulation of arousal and reactions to stress. Overall, the research supports both overreactivity and lack of proper feedback regulation to the hypothalamic-pituitary-adrenal system.

No Safe Place

The more one judges, the less one loves.
Honoré de Balzac

When the rest of us are resting, daydreaming, or just reflecting on our experiences, people with BPD demonstrate hypermetabolism in the motor cortex, anterior cingulate, temporal pole, left superior parietal gyrus, and right superior frontal gyrus. They also show decreased frontal activity, frontolimbic connectivity, deficits in cortical inhibition, and abnormalities in critical network connectivity. Deficits in metabolism are also seen in the precuneus parietal lobes and posterior cingulate regions that contribute to the inner experience of self and autobiographical memory.

Taken together, these data and the reports of our clients suggest that they lack a safe internal space to which they can retreat. In fact, relaxing may flood them with painful thoughts and emotions too difficult to bear. Although capable of mentalizing their experiences, their thoughts are often distorted by negative and frightening information. These patients often report escalating anxiety and fear, to the point where they are crawling out of their skin. They often engage in risk-taking behavior, substance abuse, and inflicting harm on themselves attempting to escape their pain and fear. The inability to be alone may be due to the fact that these clients have to rely on others to distract them from their inner worlds, which trigger their **abandonment panic**.

Definition: Abandonment Panic

Abandonment panic in an adult with BPD can be thought of as a flashback to emotions of an infant who can't find his mother. He is overwhelmed with anxiety, panic, and fear for his life. There is nowhere to run because the fear is coming from within; still, the desire to escape is overwhelming. These experiences and the self-injurious behavior they trigger are stored in subcortical and right-hemisphere-based brain regions.

For clients with borderline-type behaviors, abandonment cues trigger a posttraumatic flashback of life-threatening proportions. Patients become consumed and overwhelmed with fear and desperately try to stop their pain by any means possible. This is one reason why they have a catastrophic reaction to separation and are so afraid of being alone. The most salient indication for the therapist of being with a borderline individual is feeling attacked, inadequate, and in emotional danger—because this is exactly what the client feels. This is where your countertransference can be a useful tool. Our reactions to such clients may be our best window to the chaotic emotional world of their early childhood.

One of the central tools of the psychotherapist is the interpretation, a statement that attempts to make unconscious material conscious. Borderline clients often demonstrate extreme negative emotional reactions to interpretations and may become enraged or violent, or leave the consulting room. They lack the ability to reflect on their own thoughts, making self-monitoring across emotional states almost impossible. Decompensation in the face of interpretations may reflect a rapid shift from frontal to subcortical (amygdala) dominance, manifesting in an emotional storm and functional regression.

The leverage in these situations, as in other posttraumatic reactions, is to expand the neural ensemble to include systems involved in conscious processing and left to right hemisphere inhibition.

Establishing a warm human connection serves to downregulate amygdala activation and panic, which, in turn, allows for left cortical processing to become activated. My presence and ability to stay focused on the client's feelings despite all distractions allows me to be a soothing presence. Once this attunement is established, the goal is to simultaneously activate left frontal neural networks through the use of language that allows for self-reflection and inhibition of subcortical and right-hemisphere networks. The addition of these networks to the ensemble of the flashback allows the experience to be "corticalized" and eventually brought under conscious control. Without the participation of these networks, the client is a passive victim of implicit memories.

The human connection allows three important and interrelated events: (1) a downregulation of arousal and panic via connection; (2) the activation of left frontal networks via language that serve to inhibit subcortical and right-hemisphere affect arousal; (3) therapeutic interaction here is the addition of a cortical component to a primarily subcortical process.

Self-Disgust

I think everyone struggles with self-love.

Philip Seymour Hoffman

Closely associated with the fear of abandonment is the experience of core shame (Chapter 8). In essence, core shame is the conscious elaboration of abandonment experiences. Any real or imagined slight activates the memory of abandonment and the fear of death, which develops as life's central theme. Worthlessness and the inevitability of abandonment and death are deeply known, utterly true, and tragically certain. It is a sentence that has yet to be carried out—a lifetime spent on death row—always vigilant for the sound of a key rattling in the lock.

Clients with BPD seem to experience core shame at a more intense level than others. Self-awareness triggers a feeling of self-disgust, often leading them to describe themselves as gross, pathetic losers. They often stay away from others because they can't imagine that others don't see them the same way they see themselves.

The psychodynamic interpretation of this disgust is based on an internalization of how they experienced their parents experiencing them. It may also be related to the early development of the social brain, specifically the insula and anterior cingulate cortices, which controls our sense of disgust related to taking in food. Perhaps, for these clients, their earliest experience of mother was of disgust for them. That would certainly parallel the deep emotional connection between food and family, especially mother.

Neuroscience Corner: The Insula and Anterior Cingulate Cortices

Organized like maps of the body, the insula cortex and the anterior cingulate connect primitive bodily states with the experience and expression of emotion, behavior, and cognition and are involved with mediating the gamut of emotions from disgust to love. The insula participates in the organization and experience of our core sense of self in space and our ability to distinguish between self and others. Interestingly, both the insula and anterior cingulate become activated when subjects are asked to recall behavior for which they felt ashamed.

Disgust is a very primitive emotion shaped by evolution to make us reflexively retreat from potential danger—usually contamination from food, blood, and bodily damage. The gag and vomit reflexes are triggered to get toxic substances out of our bodies and have been generalized to corpses and blood, which puts us on guard and makes us wary of both potential predators and toxic microorganisms. Overall, the emotion of disgust is one of avoidance and expulsion, either from the body or from one's personal space.

The possibility exists that the early experiences of borderline individuals may lead them to pair the sense of self with disgust, perhaps through feeling pushed away or abandoned, or seeing a look of disgust on a caretaker's face, like a response to poisonous or rotten food. One study found that women diagnosed with BPD or PTSD had greater "disgust sensitivity" and were prone to be disgusted with their self-image. When women with BPD recalled memories of childhood, they also tend to show disgusted facial expressions.

Given their roles in emotion and early development, the insula and anterior cingulate cortex may play a central role in our ability to relate to ourselves and others. In the context of secure attachment, feelings of love and positive bodily states may become linked with the organization of self-awareness. If the infant experiences neglect or abuse, or sees disgust or despair in the eyes of caretakers, disgust and expulsion may come to be associated with the experience of self. For these individuals who would certainly be candidates to develop core shame, self-awareness would trigger despair, rage, and self-loathing.

Based on all of these clinical and research findings, it is entirely possible that what we call borderline personality disorder is a form of PTSD triggered by disturbances of early attachment experiences. For these individuals, the primitive executive systems organized around the amygdala continue to organize their experience and navigate their way through life. This manner of being may have been perfectly adaptive to tribal life in our deep history but is no longer adequate to deal with the complex social and cognitive challenges of modern life. Understanding the victims of early attachment trauma in this way might lead to more humane and less critical perceptions of what we call borderline personality disorder and to treatments that are better matched to their struggles.

CHAPTER 14

The Power of
Coherent Narratives

An attack upon our ability to tell stories is not just censorship—
it is a crime against our nature as human beings.
Salman Rushdie

HUMANS GATHERED TO share stories far back into pre-history. This impulse to gather and gossip has served to maintain and transmit culture across individuals, generations, and cultures. Be it tales of ancestors, strategies for successful hunting, or to just pass the time with friends and family, the stories of tribes have served to strengthen relationships, coordinate group behavior, and advance the development of abstract thinking.

Thus, our social brains coevolved with storytelling, narrative structure, and the tales of heroic journeys still told throughout the world. Stories are, in fact, so ubiquitous in human experience that we hardly notice their existence. Just think of all the energy we invest in gossiping across every new medium of communication. This constant information exchange is likely a large part of our adaptation capacity that allowed *Homo habilis* to survive dramatic climate changes while many other lines of primate evolution became extinct.

As a medium for the articulation of personal experience and shared values, stories connect families, tribes, and nations, generate culture, and link us to a group mind. These connections, in turn, support the functioning and well-being of each individual brain. It is no coincidence that storytelling is a cornerstone of what we call the talking cure—psychotherapy. It is very likely that our brains have been able to become as complex as they are precisely because of the power of narratives to integrate both our brains and social groups.

Culture and Identity

The universe is made of stories, not of atoms.
Muriel Rukeyser

Stories are a central aspect of individual identity and in many ways we come to live the stories we, and others, tell about us. They describe our experiences, strengths, and aspirations as well as our past failures and negative self-attributions. As children we are told who we are, what is important to us, and what we are capable of by our families. We then take these stories out into the world and continue to edit them with teachers, peers, and cultural input. The impact of stories on the formation of self-identity makes them powerful tools in the creation and maintenance of the self. Positive self-narratives aid in emotional security while negative ones perpetuate low self-esteem, anxiety, and pessimism. In this way, our stories become blueprints for our future.

Every culture has stories, myths, and fables born before the written word and shared via storytelling and song. The Vedic song poems of ancient India were memorized, sung, and passed on by a class of scholars dedicated to the preservation of ancient wisdom. The accumulation and advancement of knowledge was completely dependent on the compulsion to hear and tell stories and the brain's ability to remember. This is probably why we possess a limitless capacity for remembering stories and songs while it is often hard to remember what we had for lunch. This is because stories have been far more important historically to our survival than remembering specific details.

It has always been the job of the elders to tell stories, passing them on to the younger members of the tribe. A wonderful window to this deep history is reflected in the way elders and children relate to stories. As people grow older, they have a tendency to tell more stories from longer ago, as if the distant past becomes increasingly salient with age. Now think of who likes to hear the same stories again and again and again in exactly the same way. In fact, they will even correct you if you get a word or fact incorrect. If you guessed young children, you are right. They demand that you tell them the same story every night for days, weeks, or months before they are ready to move on to the next one. Children do naturally what ancient Indian scholars turned into their life's work—remembering ancient wisdom.

What we are likely witnessing in these parallel processes is a preprogrammed process in both adult and child to transfer the stories, knowledge, and wisdom across the generations. This impulse near the beginning and end of life to repeatedly tell and listen to stories appears to be a lock-and-key mechanism of the intergenerational transfer of knowledge.

Hemispheric and Interpersonal Integration

If history were taught in the form of stories, it would never be forgotten.

Rudyard Kipling

As the human brain evolved, an increasing number of specialized neural networks emerged to handle the vast amount of information required for complex social interactions, abstract thinking, and imagination. Keeping this growing bureaucracy of neural networks integrated, balanced, and running smoothly became ever more challenging. The increasing complexity that eventually allowed for the emergence of storytelling also assisted in keeping the government of neural systems running smoothly.

The structure of any story contains two basic elements: the first is a series of events grounded in the passage of time, and the second is some emotional experience giving the story meaning. In order to tell a good story, the linear linguistic processing of the left hemisphere must be integrated with the centers in the right hemisphere that process sensory and emotional information. Thus, a coherent and meaningful narrative provides the executive brain with the best template and strategy for the oversight and coordination of the functions of brain and mind across the two hemispheres. In fact, the understandability of our narratives is related to the quality of our attachments, self-esteem, and emotional regulation.

Stories not only integrate and connect our cerebral hemispheres, they also connect us to each other. Have you ever noticed what happens in talking to a group, when you transition from talking about facts to telling a personal, emotional story? Eye contact locks in, distractions decrease, and a series of expressions on the faces of listeners reflects the emotions within the story. Listening to stories is a form of learning that goes back long before the invention of reading, writing, or arithmetic, containing all of the elements to stimulate neuroplasticity and learning.

Emotional Regulation

> *Memory is the way we keep telling ourselves our stories—and telling other people a somewhat different version of our stories.*
> Alice Munro

During the first 18 months of life, the brain's right hemisphere experiences a sensitive period of development as the physical and emotional aspects of interpersonal experience begin to take shape. These early experiences, vital to our future relationships and emotional health, are stored in systems of unconscious, implicit memory. As the left hemisphere enters its sensitive period during the middle of the second year, spoken language slowly begins to take shape and integrates with the emotional aspects of communication already organized in the right hemisphere. As the language centers mature, words are joined together to make meaningful sentences.

By four to five years old, the brain has matured to the point where words and feelings can begin to be linked in meaningful ways. Putting feelings into words and using them as a component of ongoing experience contributes to the ability to regulate anxiety and fear. Putting feelings into words and sharing them with others is an ability modeled and shaped by the skills of those around us. Parents who don't talk to their children about feelings deprive them of a valuable source of emotional regulation.

Having a conscious narrative of our experience helps us remember where we have come from, where we are, and where we are going. In other words, our stories ground us in the present, within the flow of our histories, and provide a direction for the future. This linear blueprint helps us to avoid feeling lost in an external present while reducing anxiety triggered by uncertainty. Within the brain, the cognitive processes involved in creating a narrative activate frontal functioning that downregulates amygdala activation. Essentially, having a narrative that creates a sense of control puts us in a state of mind that prepares us to think while reducing our anxiety and fear. Believing you are an efficacious person stimulates frontal activation that makes you a more efficacious person. There actually is power in positive thinking.

Having your clients write about their experiences in diaries and journals supports the same top-down emotional regulation as telling their story to others. Journaling increases a sense of well-being and reduces things like physical symptoms, physician visits, and missing work. Putting our thoughts and feelings into words through stories and journaling is also believed to stimulate prefrontal cortical areas that inhibit amygdala activation. These changes in neural activity result in a cascade of positive physiological, behavioral, and emotional effects, such as boosting immunological health (greater T-helper response, natural killer cell activity, and hepatitis B antibody levels) and lowering heart rate.

Secure Attachment and Integrated Narratives

Stories in families are colossally important. . . .
Knowing them is proof of belonging.
Salman Rushdie

Narratives begin to be co-constructed in parent-child talk during the first year and continue throughout life. When verbal interactions include references to sensations, feelings, behaviors, and knowledge, they provide a medium through which the child's brain is able to integrate the various aspects of experience and the array of different neural networks that process them. For example, the optimal organization of autobiographical memory, which includes input from multiple neural networks, enhances self-awareness while increasing our ability to solve problems, cope with stress, and maintain our connections with others.

From primitive tribes to modern families, coconstructed narratives are at the core of human groups. Group participation in narrating shared experiences organizes memories, embeds them within a social context, and assists in linking feelings, actions, and others to the self. As mentioned earlier, the repetition of stories also helps children to develop and practice recall abilities and influences and shapes their memories through relationships. This mutual shaping of memory between children and adults can serve both positive and negative ends. Positive outcomes include teaching the importance of accurate memory, imparting cultural values, and shaping the child's self-image. Negative outcomes include the weaving of the caretakers' traumas and prejudices into the children's narratives. When caretakers are unable to tolerate certain emotions, those emotions will be excluded from their narratives or shaped into distorted but more acceptable forms. In this way, the narratives of children will come to reflect the parents' unconscious editorial choices. Whatever is excluded from the child's narrative will be more difficult to process and comprehend in the years to come. This is one mechanism through which we pass our unresolved issues to our children. At its extreme, parents can be so overwhelmed by the emotions related to unresolved trauma that their narratives become disjointed and incoherent. There also appears to be a causal relationship among the complexity of a child's narratives, the nature of their self-talk, and their attachment security.

Securely attached children generally engage in self-talk during toddlerhood and more spontaneous self-reflective remarks at age six. They tend to make comments about their thinking process and their ability to remember things about their history. These processes of mind, which insecurely attached children often lack, reflect the utilization of narratives in the development of self-identity and metacognition. As you might expect, children who are abused are usually insecurely attached and less able to think about their thinking or engage in self-reflection. This suggests that the ability to reflect on the self and one's thoughts plays a role in emotional regulation, memory integration, and executive functioning.

The Capacity to Be

> *Beware the barrenness of a busy life.*
> Socrates

Many men that I've worked with wake up in the middle of their lives feeling like strangers to themselves. Often, they have spent their lives living up to the expectations of others but never took the time to explore their own desires, passions, or interests. Perhaps this is part of midlife crisis, but it feels deeper to me. It isn't the recognition that you aren't young anymore; it's the recognition that you no longer feel alive. It might be that you were tracked to medical or law school when you were 12 and never explored your interests in music or the arts. Or you got married and started to have children in your early 20s, and there was never the time, money, or conscious space to think about what might be important beyond taking care of other people.

Years ago, I was planning a vacation with a group of friends to Moorea, a small island a few miles south of Tahiti. We started talking about it in January, and by May, we had our reservations booked for August. As the time approached, one after another of my companions backed out. I considered canceling myself, but I needed a vacation. So on August first, I found myself boarding the nine-hour flight on my own.

For this story to make sense, you have to know that, up until this point in my life, I was never a good or willing vacationer. I generally worked seven days a week on one project or another and measured the quality of my life by accomplishments. If I wasn't working with clients, I was fixing the house, writing papers, reading, or being productive in some other way. The only time I realized that I had forgotten to take time off was when I would develop an intractable headache that signaled a need for a break.

When I got off the plane in Tahiti, I took a cab to the dock and boarded a ferry bound for Moorea. Once on Moorea, a bus that circled the island dropped me off in front of my hotel. I checked in, found my little hut on the beach, unpacked my things, put on my bathing suit, and sat on the deck to stare at the ocean. After 30 seconds, I began to get fidgety and wondered what there was to do. I went to the front desk to ask for a suggestion, and the local girls all agreed that the tour of the pineapple factory was by far the most interesting thing to do there. Really, it was the only tourist attraction on the island. So I went, saw how pineapples were processed and packaged, and half an hour later was back at the hotel. So I went back to my hut and sat back down on the deck to relax and stare at the ocean.

I had landed in Tahiti at 4 A.M., arrived in Moorea by 7 A.M., was at the pineapple factory by 9, and back to the hotel by 11. It had been a very long day and I still had a while to wait for lunch. I felt like I was in a time distortion zone where every minute was an hour long. After a few more minutes (hours) of relaxing, I felt like I might go crazy, so I walked over to the bar to get a mai tai with a little umbrella in it. Sensing my desperation, the bartender may have added a splash of extra alcohol, because it almost immediately put me to sleep. Awakening a few hours later with a sunburn and a different kind of headache, I slowly struggled to regain my wits. I realized that back home, the days raced by as I tried to complete my lists of things to do. In my day-to-day life, it seemed like breakfast came every 10 minutes. It was now almost three o'clock on the day of my arrival, and the day felt like an eternity. I felt as if I had already had enough vacation, thank you very much. What was I going to do for the next three weeks?

One advantage of being a therapist is that, in times like these, you eventually remember that you have an unconscious. Next, you remember that when you feel like you are losing your mind, some emotion is getting activated that you don't understand. The next thing to do is to consider the feelings, free associate, and be open to whatever comes to mind.

In the face of this home remedy, my first association was to my childhood, and I began to remember how slowly time appeared to pass. I remembered how long summer vacation seemed to be, how long it felt from Thanksgiving to Christmas, and how endless Sunday afternoons visiting with relatives seemed to be. I shuttled to the present moment and realized that the three weeks ahead of me felt like a vast expanse of time. And I began to realize that time is a matter of being emotionally present. One of the prices I was paying for being so "productive" was that I had forgotten how to be. It turned out that I had such a good time on my vacation that I returned the following year.

The Hero's Journey

A hero is an ordinary individual who finds the strength to persevere and endure in spite of overwhelming obstacles.
Christopher Reeve

What makes for a good story, and why do we feel compelled to watch movies like *Pretty Woman* or *A Few Good Men* over and over again? There is a formula, and any screenwriting class can teach it to you. Every story needs a hero with whom the audience can identify, a good hero simultaneously facing an external challenge and struggling with some inner wound that causes persistent pain. For the characters played by both Richard Gere and Tom Cruise, this pain came from estrangement from their fathers—a common dilemma of adolescent males who face the challenge of becoming an adult without the guidance and support of a nurturing father. Not surprisingly, this is my story and likely drives my fascination with both films. The challenge for Gere is to face his vulnerability, while for Cruise, it is living up to his father's reputation. Does Gere have the guts to fall in love with Julia Roberts? Does Cruise have what it takes to go toe-to-toe with Jack Nicholson?

At first, the hero avoids or fails the challenge, leading him to question his ability to succeed. The challenge is repeatedly questioned and even rejected before it is eventually accepted. During the journey, the hero leaves behind old definitions of self and travels into uncharted territory before discovering his own meaning and place in the world. Some inner transformation takes place that allows him to face his demons, succeed in his worldly challenge, and solidify a new and expanded adult identity, which now includes previously unintegrated thoughts, behaviors, and emotions.

This narrative structure, seen in stories around the world and throughout time, has also been called the myth of the hero by Joseph Campbell. It is a core theme of ancient mythology, contemporary literature, and most children's stories. It is the story of the adolescent struggle toward adulthood, the overcoming of fear and trauma, and personal transformation and redemption. The universality of this story is likely the result of the commonality of brain evolution, shared developmental challenges, and the fundamental emotional similarities of human development. Despite our cultural differences, all humans share the fight for growth, survival, and actualization. Below, I outline some common aspects of the heroic journey in more detail.

Key Aspects of the Hero's Journey

The Journey Begins

The hero has an outer challenge to be faced and an inner brokenness to be healed.

Accomplishing these goals requires taking a journey to new and unknown places.

The journey offers a promise of growth and redemption.

The Challenge

The present system and the current self are insufficient and cannot save you.

You must venture forth beyond the safe and familiar confines of your life and beliefs.

Past rules will be broken in the cause of finding what can only be found elsewhere.

Finding the Guide

The guide acknowledges and respects the brokenness and shame that lurk in the hero's shadows.

The guide sees beyond the hero's limitations.

The guide presents an invitation and a challenge to take the heroic journey.

Attaching to the Guide

The guide has something and believes the hero can have it too.

The hero becomes aware that the guide sees something real in the world and in him.

The hero comes to gradually share the guide's vision.

The Heroic Discovery

Limitations exist only in the mind.

Confronting fear and pain are gateways to new worlds.

Power is discovered in vulnerability; freedom is found in commitment.

Carl Jung said that the answers to our most important questions are to be found in the shadow. The shadow is the repository of our pain and shame—the horrors of our families and the demons of our inner lives. Because you can't completely banish the shadow, you must learn to develop a relationship with it. If the shadow can be acknowledged and included in the therapeutic relationship, the therapist becomes transformed from a source of information to a guide on the path to wisdom. Wisdom is a form of knowledge delivered with compassion and shaped in a manner that helps the seeker to heal and grow. Put in a slightly different way, wisdom is knowledge in the service of others.

In order for therapists to become guides, they need to be familiar with their own shadows, which allows them to identify, approach, and confront their clients' inner demons. Like shamans, therapists have to have a clear vision so that their client can come to believe that they see something real that they can share in. The message is, "I know something you don't know, something you don't have, but I am committed to sharing it with you and helping you along on your journey." Sometimes, therapists need to tell their clients stories of what is possible, stories that connect us to the unconscious, our tribal histories, and to potential futures. These stories can become the road map to a better future.

Therapists have to be able to acknowledge the pain, suffering, hypocrisy, and lack of fairness in the world. They have to have faced it for themselves and come out on the other side with their own sense of purpose and meaning in order to be a guide for someone else. Therapists also have to acknowledge their own shadow and make it a part of the therapy. A therapist invites clients to take a journey out of the narrow confines of their lives into a new world beyond the limitations of their neighborhood, family, culture, and current narrative.

Everyone has a story. In the absence of self-awareness, our story is a simple chronology of events and our judgments about them. Psychotherapy is a metacognitive vantage point with the potential to add self-awareness to our story. This bit of objective distance provides us with the ability to think about our story, reflect on our choices, and consider editing some of the outcomes. Sometimes you have to make some suggestions about alternative narrative arcs and outcomes to get them started. Would my family really disown me if I followed my own dreams? Would it kill my father if I told him the truth about who I am? Is there a possibility that I could be successful and happy?

As therapists, we hope to guide our clients to the realization that they are more than a character in a story dictated by external circumstances. Often, a large portion of a client's story has been unconsciously imposed by past generations of their families. What makes it especially hard to edit is that much of this origin is unconscious. We would love to instill in our clients that they can make choices, follow their passions, and become the author of a new story—their story. The narrative process allows us to separate story from self. It's like taking off your shirt to patch a tear and then putting it back on. When we evolved the capacity to examine our narratives and see them as one option among many, we also gained the ability to edit and modify our lives.

CHAPTER 15

Pain Is Inevitable; Suffering Is Optional

We are healed from suffering only by experiencing it to the full.
Marcel Proust

PAIN AND LIFE are one. There is the pain of childbirth and the pain of learning that you cannot protect your child from pain. Later comes the pain of growing old, dying, and leaving your children behind. And this is the best-case scenario. How we deal with life's pain is a reflection of the depth of our inner world, our resilience, and a core element of our character.

After being traumatized by his first encounters with sickness, aging, and death, Buddha grew despondent and left his home in search of a teacher. He had become convinced that life was suffering and searched for a path to liberation. What he discovered two millennia ago is now being rediscovered by modern science—while pain is inevitable, suffering is a product of the mind. This means that we can use our minds to change how we experience our lives. In my words, we can use our minds to change our brains.

Not many of us are on our way to becoming enlightened beings. I'm certainly not about to give up my flat-screen TV and ice cream to search for truth. However, there are aspects of Buddha's teachings that can benefit us in the comfort of our privileged lives. From my perspective, the most important is that while pain is inevitable, it is also transitory. We can grin, bear it, and wait it out. I remember watching the World Trade Center burning and wondering if my oldest friend was trapped in his top-floor office. But I also knew, even as I was being traumatized by what I was seeing, even as I imagined my friend choking on smoke and trying to help others stay calm, that life would go on, that people would forget, and that a new generation would come along, who never had the twin towers as fixtures on their daily horizon.

What Buddha taught us is that long after our pain has subsided, suffering can become a habit of the brain and program of the mind. We are capable of becoming attached to our losses, grudges, and slights, and we turn transitory pain into a lifetime of hurt. This is an insight that has to be discovered again and again by each generation of therapists across all theoretical perspectives. So while it is clear that life contains much pain, it doesn't have to lead to unending suffering. I have personal proof of this because, while my childhood was characterized by considerable suffering, my adult life is not—even though there has been plenty of pain.

Niagara Falls

> But if thought corrupts language, language can also corrupt thought.
> George Orwell

As a small boy during the 1960s, I noticed that my grandparents never took vacations together. I asked my grandmother why, and she said that my grandfather hadn't asked her to vacation with him since World War II, when she had said something that hurt his feelings. That made me curious, because my grandpa was as tough as they came, drove a big truck, and carried iron bathtubs up flights of stairs—I couldn't imagine my sweet little grandmother hurting his feelings. Here is the story as it was told to me.

As a teenager during the 1920s, my grandmother went to a vaudeville show with her girlfriends and heard a joke that she found quite funny. One person asked another, "Would you like to go to Niagara Falls for the weekend?" and the other responded, "Is that place still running?" Despite the fact that my grandmother was not the joke-telling type, she found this one particularly funny, and it lodged in some corner of her brain for future use.

Fast forward a decade or two—my grandparents and their children (my father among them) are sitting at the dinner table. My grandfather spent his days cleaning and repairing ships returning from combat in the North Atlantic. I can only imagine how little money they had, how grueling and difficult his work was, and how much of a stretch it must have been for him to pop the question to her: "Would you like to go to Niagara Falls for a little vacation?"—a wonderful gesture on his part.

The words "Niagara Falls" triggered the memory of this joke in my grandmother's mind, and she responded to my grandfather with the punch line, "Is that place still running?" I suspect she said it in the same sarcastic and offhanded way the seasoned comedian had said it all those years ago. My grandmother's expectation was to get a good laugh and then discuss the trip—she would have loved to go. To her surprise, my grandfather's response was to feel belittled and ashamed. He got up from the table and went to bed. Neither of them ever brought it up again, nor did they ever go on that or any other vacation. They possessed neither the courage to confront their feelings nor the skills to discuss them.

So what does this sad little story from my family's past have to do with pain and suffering? I think it is an excellent example of how a moment of pain can become a lifetime of suffering. My grandfather's momentary pain was converted by both of their brains and minds into a lifetime of distance within their relationship. Had the pain been expressed, my grandmother's statement explained, apologies been exchanged, they could have had a nice vacation and a better relationship. But because both of their brains triggered fear and withdrawal, nothing was discussed, and their minds were left with constructing the other person's intentions based on their respective histories of loss and rejection. I suspect all relationships have minor disasters like this that decrease intimacy and joy.

Getting Back on the Horse That Threw You

> *You yourself, as much as anyone in the universe,*
> *deserve your love and affection.*
> Buddha

When I was growing up, "getting back on the horse that threw you" was shorthand for facing fears and not letting them guide and limit your life. All these years later, I read that a powerful correlate of therapeutic success is the reduction of approach anxiety—same thing. The way not to be controlled by fear is to approach what you are afraid of in order to retrain your amygdala and sympathetic nervous system not to get activated in the face of what they have paired with danger. In a parallel process, the best way to combat pain is through a combination of anger and vulnerability, the two things that shame drives us to avoid.

The way to minimize suffering is to approach pain and create a way of understanding and sharing it with others. If you avoid the challenges you are afraid of and survive another day, the fears become more deeply ingrained in your nervous system. Put in another way, withdrawal gets reinforced within our brains as an overarching survival strategy. This is the essence of exposure therapy. This is why clients do better when they are able to approach what makes them anxious and afraid. These experiments in courage, both in and out of therapy, are a central mechanism of brain change.

So what could my grandparents have done during World War II to avert half a century of hard feelings? My grandfather could have said that he was excited about the trip and expected her to be excited and happy as well. He also could have said that the unexpected joke hurt his feelings. My grandmother could have apologized, told the story from her girlhood, poked him on the top of his head (as she always did), and said that she would love to go on a trip to Niagara Falls. Of course, they both lacked a language for their feelings, and negative emotions only triggered stronger defenses, attacks, or more dramatic withdrawals.

In contrast, when pain is met by emotional numbing, it generalizes across all emotions and makes life far less enjoyable. When the pain is numbed, all feelings are numbed and you are left with a dead relationship and a dead life, so the applications of Buddha's message to therapy are clear:

1. Reframe your avoidance of anxiety and fear into curiosity. Be an emotion detective and figure out what is beneath the fear. If we go down a layer or two, below the anger, resentment, and shame, sooner or later we all get to a fear of abandonment. Realize that our brains feed all sorts of information to our minds—a good deal of which is misinformation. It is up to us to learn to tell the good from the bad. But remember, sometimes a cigar is just a cigar.

2. Move toward the broken places. Embrace pain sooner rather than later; move toward it, let it wash over you, feel grief, wail, scream, and say what's on your mind. Get really good at approaching pain and learn as early in life as possible that you will survive. I realize this may seem counterintuitive, but our intuitions, like our thoughts, are fallible.

3. Get enraged! Allow yourself to become as angry as you are able at your brain for feeding you misinformation. If you have a brain and mind that constantly tell you that you are inferior, worthless, and unlovable, tell them to get lost. Learn the ways in which your brain converts pain into suffering and insist that it stop. If your brain and mind are not your friends, stop taking their advice.

4. Share your feelings in as respectful a way as you are able. If your feelings involve other people and they are still alive, there is an opportunity to salvage or build a relationship. Start opening up. It will be hard, of course, and you will not do it perfectly. There is no perfection to be attained and no final resting point. Relationships are an endless river of energy moving toward an invisible sea.

What's Wrong With Me?

Beware of false knowledge; it is more dangerous than ignorance.
George Bernard Shaw

Stan walked into our first meeting ready to go. As he sat down, he began, "Hey Doc, do you remember the one about the frog and the pot of boiling water?" Before I could reply, Stan continued, "If you drop a frog into boiling water, it panics and jumps out—smart frog! But if you put a frog in cool water and raise the temperature slowly, you have dinner—if you like frog. I guess you could say that because the frog doesn't notice the small changes, he wakes up dead." A big smile spread across his broad face.

I had talked with Stan a week earlier, when he had complained of feeling lost. He was careful to distinguish it from depression, which he had experienced early in life. At 60, he was married with three children, had a successful financial consulting practice, and "on paper" (as he put it) had a good life. There was no particular thing he could point to as the cause of his unease—he loved his wife; his kids were doing well; he had a few good friends he saw on a regular basis—but for some reason, none of it seemed to matter anymore. "I think I'm the frog. I have a sense that I forgot to pay attention to something important, and then I forgot to remember. I'm going through the motions of my life, but the spark is gone."

We sat in silence together as I let what he had said wash over me. I began to get a physical sense of his "lostness" that grew into an emptiness in my chest, a feeling of deflation, followed by sadness—I felt as if I could melt into my chair. Stan looked at my face, saw my sadness, and went deeper. "I feel guilty about saying this, but with everything I have, I still feel like there is something missing: I don't feel ungrateful, just lost." I now said my first words: "Have you ever had this kind of feeling before?" I could tell from his eyes that he had mentally left the room and was watching a scene from his past.

Stan seemed to suddenly become aware of my presence and embarrassed for having left me alone. He began to describe his journey. "When you asked me about having this feeling before, I was snapped back to a time when my father left us when I was seven. I was standing next to a bookcase and listening to my mother yell at him over the phone. I didn't exactly understand what was happening or what it meant, but I do remember feeling as if I was floating in space. I know it sounds crazy, but I think I felt like we were all going to die. I felt like I was falling into a dream."

It didn't seem like Stan needed to be rescued, so I sat with him and watched the waves of emotion cross his face. I stayed grounded in the feelings; I wanted him to know I was going on this journey with him and that he didn't have to worry about taking care of me. As I sat there, I reflected on Stan's feeling that his mother and siblings would die as a consequence of his father's absence. Stan didn't realize that while his family probably wasn't at risk, for most of human prehistory, abandonment by the father would mean death to his wife and children. I wondered whether all young primates retain this memory within the primitive regions of our brains.

"A memory from 50 years ago still has power over me," he reflected. "But how could that have anything to do with what I'm feeling now? Isn't it just a coincidence?" "Possibly," I said. "Time will tell. Let's see if you have any other memories or associations to this feeling of lostness. Just allow yourself to have whatever thoughts come to mind and share them with me when you are ready." As we sat together, I could tell Stan was searching his mind for memories when his body jolted. "Another time was when I broke up with my girlfriend before I left for the East Coast to do my MBA. I knew we weren't a good fit, and I certainly didn't want to have a long-distance relationship, but I remember driving across the country, feeling like I was driving off the edge of the earth with that same empty feeling."

"Both of the experiences you describe involve abandonment and loss. In the first one, your father left you. In the second you left a girlfriend. How long had you been together?" "Six years, three months, and seventeen days—I still remember." Stan added proudly, "I also remember that even though I broke up with her, I felt betrayed when I left for school, like she had broken up with me. I guess I wanted her to fight for the relationship and not let me go. Instead, she said she understood and wished me luck." I reflected for a while and eventually said, "Maybe it doesn't matter who leaves whom; the child in us always feels abandoned when attachments are broken."

A few sessions later, he came in with a discovery he was anxious to share. He had experienced a strong bout of the lost feeling again. He had been sitting alone in his chair at midnight watching TV when the image of driving off the edge of the earth returned to him. "I asked myself again and again, why now, why now, why am I having this feeling again—and then it dawned on me." Stan had spent the day helping his youngest daughter get ready to leave for college—helping her pack, looking at maps to help plan her drive, finding rest stops along the way of her 400-mile journey up the California coast.

This was the last of his three children to leave home—his 30-year role of being a day-to-day father would soon be over. Stan seemed sad to realize the source of his emptiness. "I never thought that it would be related to Crissie leaving for college. I was fine when her two older brothers left for school and I feel proud of her for going to a great college. It's a completely natural thing. What a messed-up brain I have!" I reassured him that there was nothing messed up with his mind except the fact that in addition to having been traumatized by being abandoned by his father, his brain was reacting naturally to loss. I told him, "Even though separations make sense to our rational minds, our primitive brains are still hurt—this is not sickness; it's just how we're wired."

"In addition to this, you are transitioning out of a role that you have been in every day for the last three decades. Your kids have been your emotional ground zero for half of your adult life. You have to expect to have a reaction." "There is more to it than that," Stan said. "As my wife and I focused more and more on the kids, we let our relationship fade away. I'm not even sure we know or like each other anymore, and I'm afraid that once Crissie leaves, she won't have any reason to stay with me anymore." The first phase of therapy ended, and the second one was about to begin.

Finite and Infinite

> *Remember your dreams and fight for them.*
> Paulo Coelho

Psychotherapy isn't rocket science—it is far more complex. Rocket scientists enjoy the benefits of shutting off input from their bodies, turning off their feelings, and forgetting about their personal pasts. They have the luxury of focusing on singular processes using linear logic. They don't have to worry about their emotions biasing the principles of physics and mathematics. These parameters define both the achievements and limitations of purely scientific explorations and explanations.

Good-enough psychotherapy requires that we reach inside and become open to the limitations of our knowledge and try to account for the naturally occurring distortions of our minds and brains. We use science, but it is one of many frames of reference that therapists have to employ each hour.

We can't protect each other from the pain of life. There are so many times in life when there are no words—sitting in hospitals, at funerals, and even coffee shops when we are confronted with the darkness of sickness, aging, and death. Sometimes we find ourselves in these lands of deep and difficult emotions, where we enter terra incognita, where the standard statement and clichés sound hollow, where the streets have no names.

And when I go there, I go there with you. It's all I can do.
U2

Index

The Norton Series on Interpersonal Neurobiology

Louis Cozolino, PhD, Series Editor

Allan N. Schore, PhD, Series Editor, 2007–2014

Daniel J. Siegel, MD, Founding Editor

The field of mental health is in a tremendously exciting period of growth and conceptual reorganization. Independent findings from a variety of scientific endeavors are converging in an interdisciplinary view of the mind and mental well-being. An interpersonal neurobiology of human development enables us to understand that the structure and function of the mind and brain are shaped by experiences, especially those involving emotional relationships.

The Norton Series on Interpersonal Neurobiology provides cutting-edge, multidisciplinary views that further our understanding of the complex neurobiology of the human mind. By drawing on a wide range of traditionally independent fields of research—such as neurobiology, genetics, memory, attachment, complex systems, anthropology, and evolutionary psychology—these texts offer mental health professionals a review and synthesis of scientific findings often inaccessible to clinicians. The books advance our understanding of human experience by finding the unity of knowledge, or consilience, that emerges with the translation of findings from numerous domains of study into a common language and conceptual framework. The series integrates the best of modern science with the healing art of psychotherapy.